Bayesian Methods
in Health Economics

Chapman & Hall/CRC Biostatistics Series

Chapman & Hall/CRC Biostatistics Series

Chapman & Hall/CRC Biostatistics Series

Bayesian Methods in Health Economics

Gianluca Baio

University College London
London, UK

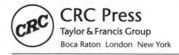

CRC Press
Taylor & Francis Group
Boca Raton London New York

CRC Press is an imprint of the
Taylor & Francis Group, an **informa** business
A CHAPMAN & HALL BOOK

CRC Press
Taylor & Francis Group
6000 Broken Sound Parkway NW, Suite 300
Boca Raton, FL 33487-2742

First issued in paperback 2022

Version Date: 2012904

ISBN 13: 978-1-03-247753-4 (pbk)
ISBN 13: 978-1-4398-9555-9 (hbk)

DOI: 10.1201/b13099

**Visit the Taylor & Francis Web site at
http://www.taylorandfrancis.com**

**and the CRC Press Web site at
http://www.crcpress.com**

To Marta and XX (or XY — it really doesn't matter. But come quickly, will you?!)

Contents

Preface

Health economics is a relatively new discipline, essentially characterised by the integration of different expertise and perspectives. Clearly, the clinical aspect is fundamental and the clinical background plays a basic role in the definition of any health economic evaluation. However, in its modern incarnation health economics is effectively identified by the integration of economic models and increasingly advanced statistical techniques, particularly under the Bayesian approach.

The objective of this book is to give a specialised presentation of these techniques. The book is thought to be a manual for an advanced course in statistical methods for health economics and assumes some knowledge of statistics. Specifically, throughout the book we develop models and examples using a combination of R and WinBUGS/JAGS for the main Bayesian analysis (usually based on Markov Chain Monte Carlo).

The structure of the book is the following. In Chapter 1, which is written in collaboration with Rachael M. Hunter, we introduce the main economic concepts; among them, the important distinction between financial and economic analysis and the definition of the relevant costs for health economic evaluations. The typical outcomes are also discussed, with particular reference to the distinction between "hard" clinical outcome and measures of utility derived for example by suitable questionnaires. Then, we move on to discuss the main types of economic evaluations, focussing our attention particularly on cost-effectiveness and cost-utility analysis. Finally, we discuss basic health economic concepts such as the *Incremental Cost-Effectiveness Ratio* and its use as a measure of comparison among different interventions. Some simple examples are presented to clarify the computational aspects and the interpretation of the results.

Chapter 2 presents the fundamentals of Bayesian statistics. Particularly in this chapter, some working knowledge of statistics is assumed. First, we briefly revisit the main characteristics of the Bayesian philosophy and the meaning of subjective probability. The concept of rational decision-making in the face of uncertainty (which will be considered also in Chapter 3) is discussed before moving to parametric models. Exchangeability in its implications in the Bayesian paradigm is also touched upon before moving on to the main inferential aspects. The choice of the prior distribution and its combination with the available data into the posterior distribution are presented through a set of examples. Finally, we discuss simulation techniques (such as Monte Carlo and Markov Chain Monte Carlo) in simple terms. Although the methods are discussed in detail, with the aim of guiding the unfamiliar reader through their potential and limitations, the mathematics is kept at a relatively low level.

Chapter 3 first reviews the basic concepts underpinning the application of Bayesian decision theory. In particular, we stress the importance of the decision criterion based on the maximisation of expected utilities as an equivalent means of maximising the probability of the outcome preferred by the decision-maker. We do so briefly and keeping a very low level of the mathematics involved. Then we specialise the framework to the specific health economic evaluation. This has additional complications, e.g. the fact that the utility function needs to be specified over two relevant dimensions (costs and clinical benefits). Thus specific methods for the application of Bayesian health economic evaluation are developed. In doing this, we continuously switch between the theoretical aspects and a practical application to a relatively simple, fictional problem. Finally, we move on to define and discuss the theory and practice of probabilistic sensitivity analysis (PSA), i.e. the quantification of the impact on the decision analysis of the underlying uncertainty in the model. We consider both PSA with respect to parameter and structural uncertainty.

After having discussed in the two previous chapters much of the required theory, we then move to give a detailed account of "how to do" Bayesian analysis (in Chapter 4) and health economic evaluation (in Chapter 5). In Chapter 4, we concentrate our attention on the computational aspects of Bayesian inference, and we develop a series of worked examples combining the use of R (for pre- and post-processing of the data and the results) and JAGS to execute the Bayesian estimation.

Finally, Chapter 5 presents a few worked examples of health economic evaluations, which we develop using the tools discussed in the previous chapters. We present some of the problems typically encountered in the analysis of health economic data: the first example considers a case in which individual data are available on both cost and clinical benefit data, and we use several possible distributional assumptions to perform the cost-effectiveness analysis. In the second case, we first discuss the theoretical aspects of Bayesian hierarchical models and their use in the development of evidence synthesis models, which are particularly useful in health economics. Once a suitable decision model is specified, the relevant probability distributions to be associated with the random quantities are defined starting from empirical data retrieved from the literature, rather than from observations on individuals. Finally, the third case shows an application of Markov models, an increasingly popular methodology that is particularly effective in representing dynamically the progression of patients through a set of clinically relevant states. We show two different examples, one in which the main components of the model (i.e. the transition probabilities) are directly estimated using observed data; and the other in which they are defined as functions of suitable parameters, which is the objective of the Bayesian estimation procedure.

The final version of the book has benefitted from comments and suggestions by many friends and colleagues. Among them, I would like to mention Christian Hennig, Gareth Ambler, Marta Blangiardo, Giampiero Marra and Maurizio Filippone. Martyn Plummer, Chris Jackson and two anonymous reviewers provided me with some insightful comments, particularly on Chapter 4.

Philip Dawid has been instrumental in helping me formalise the material in Chapter 3, while Rachael Hunter has brought a much needed economist's perspective to Chapter 1.

Richard Nixon, David Wonderling and Richard Grieve kindly agreed to make available the data for §5.2; similarly, Germán Rodriguez let me use his data on birth weight which have been discussed throughout Chapter 2.

Gianni Corrao and the students of the course *Statistics for Health Economics* which I taught in the University of Milano Bicocca (Italy) have been exposed to a previous version of the material presented in the book and have helped me find a balance in the topics.

Robert Calver and Rachel Holt have been the best people I have ever worked with at Chapman & Hall — OK: they are also the only ones I have ever worked with at Chapman & Hall, but that does not take anything away from their brilliant work and continuous support!

Finally, like a proper good Italian, I should also thank my *mamma* and *babbo*. If readers shared just a fraction of their unconditional love and excitement for this book, it would change the landscape of health economics forever. Of course, I do hope that readers will have more interest in the actual contents of the book and not just in the fact that my name is on it!

GIANLUCA BAIO
London, UK

Glossary

BCEA	Bayesian cost-effectiveness analysis (R package)
BUGS	Bayesian analysis using Gibbs sampling
CBA	Cost-benefit analysis
CBR	Cost-benefit ratio
CEA	Cost-effectiveness analysis
CEAC	Cost-effectiveness acceptability curve
CI	Confidence (or credible) interval
CMA	Cost-minimisation analysis
CUA	Cost-utility analysis
DAG	Directed acyclic graph
DIC	Deviance information criterion
DRG	Diagnostic related groups
DSA	Deterministic sensitivity analysis
DT	Decision trees
EIB	Expected incremental benefit
EQ-5D	EuroQol 5 dimensions
EVPI	Expected value of (perfect) information
EVPPI	Expected value of partial (perfect) information
GP	General practitioner
HPD	Highest posterior density
IB	Incremental benefit
ICER	Incremental cost-effectiveness ratio
IGLS	Iterative generalised least square
INLA	Integrated nested Laplace approximation
ISPOR	International Society for Pharmacoeconomics and Outcomes Research
JAGS	Just another Gibbs sampler
LFI	Local financial information
MAP	Maximum a posteriori
MC	Monte Carlo
MCAR	Missing completely at random
MCMC	Markov Chain Monte Carlo
MLE	Maximum likelihood estimator
MM	Markov model
MQL	Marginal quasi-likelihood
NHS	National Health Service

NICE   National Institute for Health and Clinical Excellence
OL   Opportunity loss
PBAC   Pharmaceutical Benefits Advisory Committee
PQL   Penalised quasi-likelihood
PROM   Patient reported outcome measure
PSA   Probabilistic sensitivity analysis
PV   Present value
QALY   Quality-adjusted life years
RCT   Randomised controlled trial
REML   Restricted maximum likelihood
SA   Sensitivity analysis
SF-36   Short Form 36
SF-6D   Short Form 6 dimensions
SG   Standard gamble
TTO   Time-trade off
VI   Value of information
WTP   Willingness-to-pay

1

Introduction to health economic evaluation

This chapter was written by Rachael M. Hunter (Department of Primary Care and Population Health, UCL) and Gianluca Baio

1.1 Introduction

In recent years health economics has become an increasingly important discipline in medical research, especially with the transition from the paradigm of *evidence based medicine* to that of *translational research* (Berwick, 2005; Lean ct al., 2008), which aims at making basic research applicable in the context of real practice, and under budget constraints, in order to enhance patients' access to optimal health care.

Since the 1970s, health care services have undergone dramatic changes: increasing demand for health care has generated an increase in the number of available interventions, which have sometimes been applied regardless of considerations about the actual quality and the costs associated.

Consequently, decision-makers responsible for the provision of health care are increasingly facing critical appraisal processes of the modality in which they manage the available resources, and they need to adjust the management and the evaluation of the processes used, with respect to some measures of clinical benefit. The main reasons for the necessity of containing cost associated with health care are essentially the following:

- The progressive increase of the proportion of the "older" (above 65 years) population;

- the increase of life expectancy and of the incidence of chronic and degenerative pathologies;

- the refinement of diagnostic techniques;

- the availability of innovative health technologies and therapeutic tools associated with better clinical outcomes but also with higher costs.

In this perspective, the systematic analysis of organised data provides a fundamental contribution to the identification of economically appropriate strategies. This in turns has helped the integration between several clinical and quantitative (e.g. statistics and economics) disciplines, so much that it can be reasonably argued that *health economics* is in fact a combination of medical research, epidemiology, statistics and economics. Figure 1.1 shows this concept graphically and highlights the fact that health economics encompasses more than the mere cost evaluations.

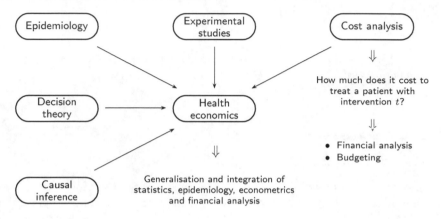

FIGURE 1.1
Health economic evaluation as the integration of different disciplines. Cost analysis only represents one side of the story.

In this chapter we present some concepts that are relevant to the definition and description of health economic evaluations. In particular we discuss the characteristics of the two dimensions along which economic evaluations are conducted: costs and clinical benefits. The latter can be defined in several different ways, each of which gives rise to a specific method of analysis. We present the main ones in §1.6. Finally, we give a first introduction to the problem of comparative evaluation of two or more health interventions, which will be discussed in more technical detail in chapters 3 and 5.

1.2   Health economic evaluation

Health economics can be formally described as the application of economic theory to *health* (defined as "a state of complete physical, mental, and social well-being and not merely the absence of disease or infirmity"; WHO, 2012) and *health care*, i.e. the diagnosis, treatment and prevention of disease and illness as delivered by medical and other practitioners.

Because the production of health care requires the use of finite resources such as labour and capital, and health can be produced (or generated), it is subject to people's needs and wants and it has an impact on welfare, both can be considered "economic goods" (Morris et al., 2007).

Health economic analysis can provide positive information about the production of health and how health care markets function, as well as normative information about the efficient and equitable production of health and health care within the finite resources available with the objective to maximise welfare.

In more general terms, however, health can be produced from economic goods other than health care, such as food, education, sanitation and housing. Further information on economic theory as it relates to health and health care can be found in Morris et al. (2007) and Folland et al. (2012).

The production of health and health care can be influenced by a range of factors, some of which are dependent on a country's government policies. These can vary widely across and within countries and can include the resources available within each country, what percentage of those resources is used to deliver health care, whether there is a state health care system and, if so, whether it is funded through taxes or social insurance, and the mix of different types of health care treatments available.

The analytical methods that will be presented throughout this book primarily address the issues of what is the best mix of health care treatments in order to maximise health. In particular, we assume the context of a developed country which already has an established health care system — resources that address reducing health inequalities, especially those experienced in developing countries, are available from the World Bank Website http://www.worldbank.org, under the topic "*Health, Nutrition and Population.*"

The issues discussed in this book are also most relevant to countries where there is some public funding of health care, be that hospitals, general health care or pharmaceuticals, and where the rationing of health care is the responsibility of a government agency.

Although still in the presence of finite resources, in private health care markets other factors that are outside the scope of this book can influence provider and consumer behaviour. Examples include moral hazard and risk management, and texts exploring the issues relating to health care funding and private health care markets include Donaldson and Gerard (2005).

Under the premise that there are finite resources available for health care, decisions need to be made on how to allocate them. For most goods and services these decisions are left up to market mechanisms as this is believed to produce the most efficient results. However, health and health care have characteristics that make them different from other goods and services and therefore, if resource allocation was left up to the markets with no government intervention, it is unlikely that the health care market would achieve the most efficient and equitable allocation of resources (Donaldson and Gerard, 2005).

As a result, governments tend to intervene by putting policies in place to control the allocation of health care. In most developed countries general practitioners (GPs) are the first point of contact with the health care system. They act as gatekeepers to the rest of the health care system, allocating resources based on need. They will only refer patients on to more expensive specialist care if they deem that care necessary for those patients. They also make decisions about what treatment(s) a patient needs and what diagnostic tests are required.

There might be a range of treatment options from which a doctor can select (e.g. different drugs to prescribe); similarly, the doctor might choose to test for other diseases that the patient might have that could benefit from earlier intervention, if identified sooner.

Since doctors are individuals with their own needs and wants and with different levels of experience and knowledge, different doctors can make different decisions about the best course of action for a given patient. Moreover, these decisions can also be influenced by other factors extrinsic to the doctor, such as financial rewards and the resources available at the moment of the decision.

In any case, once resources have been allocated to one patient, they are no longer available to treat the other individuals in the reference population. It is possible that those same resources could have achieved more (or less) benefit if made available to other patients or to different diseases, which justifies the need to perform a formal analysis in order to optmise the provision of health care in a given population.

Economic evaluation is the comparison of alternative options in terms of their *costs* and *consequences* (Drummond et al., 2005) and its purpose is to provide decision-makers with information that can help them make resource allocation decisions (Morris et al., 2007).

Historically, economic evaluation in health care has grown out of the need to make rationing decisions regarding pharmaceutical treatments paid for by tax-based health care systems. The first of these was a new level added to the Australian Pharmaceutical Benefits Advisory Committee (PBAC), the committee tasked with deciding which pharmaceutical products will be reimbursed by government funding so that the patient does not have to meet the full cost of the drug (Department of Health of the Commonwealth of Australia, 1992).

Since then, other countries have included similar methodologies in their own pharmaceutical decision-making committees, including England, Scotland and most other countries in the European Union, New Zealand and some Canadian provinces. However, each country has different requirements for pharmacoeconomic evaluations — more detailed information on geographical differences can be found on the International Society for Pharmacoeconomics and Outcomes Research (ISPOR) website http://www.ispor.org/peguidelines/index.asp.

The *National Institute for Health and Clinical Excellence* (NICE), the committee which makes decisions about which pharmaceuticals are funded within England's National Health System (NHS), recommends that economic evaluations are conducted not just for pharmaceutical products, but also as a part of other guidance including clinical, diagnostic and public health guidance (NICE, 2011).

1.2.1 Clinical trials versus decision-analytical models

Randomised controlled trials (RCTs) are a key component of the evaluation of health care interventions. They provide individual patient data where the randomisation of patients to treatment acts to reduce bias, and therefore can be used to perform head-to-head comparisons in controlled environments.

Nevertheless, the information produced by RCTs can be limited with respect to evaluating health care as delivered in the real world. This can be because the comparators in the trial do not reflect standard care available, patients are not followed up long enough to capture the full course of the illness, sample sizes are too small (especially for sub-group analysis), patient characteristics are not the same as those seen in general clinical practice or that patients are given more attention than they would generally because they are a subject in a trial (Drummond et al., 2005).

Consequently, it is advised that economic evaluations in health care take information from as many sources as possible to address some of these problems (Sculpher et al., 2006).

Decision analytical models allow for the synthesis of information across multiple sources and for the comparison of multiple options that might not have been included as part of an RCT.

Not all patients respond in the same way to treatment and therefore modelling can be used to provide information about the probability of a patient responding to a particular type of treatment. Costs and outcomes are then associated with the response variable and/or possible relevant covariates.

Values in the model can come from a combination of RCT and published information or from published information alone. A comprehensive review of the available literature should form a key component of the decision analytical model and all relevant results should be included as the omission of information can change the results of the analysis (Drummond et al., 2005).

The synthesis of information and which studies to include is not always straightforward, as some studies may not be representative of the practice being modelled. Methodologies for the synthesis of information and key considerations to make when deciding whether to include information or account for gaps in the literature are available in Drummond et al. (2005) and Briggs et al. (2006). An example of this strategy is presented in §5.3.

1.3   Cost components

1.3.1   Perspective and what costs include

The decision of which costs are included in an economic analysis is usually tailored to the requirements of the decision-makers that are the target audience of the evaluation. Which costs are included can change the result of the analysis and therefore it is important to be transparent about this aspect.

For a number of countries, health care decision making bodies only consider health care costs when assessing the *cost-effectiveness* (which we define formally in §1.6.3 and discuss in detail in Chapter 3) of an intervention. The treatment will have a specific cost associated with it, but that might be balanced by reduced disease-related hospital admissions and hence reduced cost to the overall health system. To assist decision-makers, all disease-related costs to the health system of each option should be included.

For some diseases, particularly those that will continue to impact on the patient for the rest of their life, e.g. dementia, this will mean capturing all of the health care costs of the disease for the full lifetime of the patient. On the contrary, for diseases where the impact might be over a shorter amount of time (e.g. influenza) a narrower time horizon might be more suitable.

For a number of diseases there are significant social care costs that could also be included in the analysis. This is particularly important for diseases that may result in the long term care of severely disabled patients at home or in a state institution. Whether or not to include these is dependent on how the social care services are funded and the specific question being asked.

In some instances, an analysis might include the full societal cost of a disease. This will include health and social care costs, as well as potentially extending to welfare payments for time off work, criminal justice system costs and the cost to the individual or society of unemployment, time off work or reduced performance at work. These can all be costed in different ways, which will have an impact on the final result. Therefore, it is important to be transparent about how and why these costs are included.

Family or friends of the patient might also be affected by the disease. Specifically, they may be drawn away from other activities to spend time caring for the patient. If they receive welfare or other payments from the government for this, it would be reasonable to include the resulting cost at least in some analyses.

Obviously, the cost of time caring for a family member or friend that could have been spent in employment or on leisure activities is more difficult to quantify and would only be included if a wider perspective for the analysis were being used, such as the full societal cost of the disease.

1.3.2   Sources and types of cost data

Costs can vary widely between patients, are bounded by 0, potentially have no
upper limit and hence tend to be positively skewed (Barber and Thompson,
1998; Briggs and Gray, 1998; O'Hagan and Stevens, 2001). Consequently, simple statistical models based on Normal approximations usually fail to provide
a reasonable fit to the observed data.

   Figure 1.2 shows the observed costs from a randomised trial of acupuncture
for chronic headache in primary care conducted in the UK (Wonderling et al.,
2004). Panel (a) shows a histogram of the costs for the control group (i.e.
patients treated as usual), while panel (b) presents the data for the active
treatment group, which in this case consisted of 12 acupuncture sessions from
trained physiotherapists over a three months period. As is possible to see, for
both groups the observed distribution of costs presents quite a large degree of
skewness and fit to the Normal model would be quite unsatisfactory.

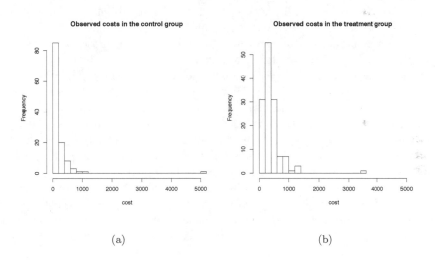

FIGURE 1.2
Histogram of the observed cost in the acupuncture RCT: panel (a) shows the
distribution for the patients in the control (treatment as usual) group, while
panel (b) shows the distribution for the patients under the active treatment.
Source: Wonderling et al. (2004).

   The usual skewness of cost data is typically due to the fact that for many
evaluations a small number of patients will cost significantly more compared
to other patients as a result of long inpatient stays or expensive interventions.
The problem is again evident in Figure 1.2, where in both groups the vast
majority of patients generates a cost lower than £1 000, with a small proportion of patients recording costs exceeding £5 000 and £3 000, respectively.

This can present additional challenges for the statistical analysis (O'Hagan and Stevens, 2003), which will be discussed in §5.2.

The type and number of different resources used can be collected in a number of ways including patient files, administrative databases, questionnaires, or the relevant literature.

The method used to collect cost data use will be dependent on whether the economic evaluation is part of a clinical trial, where access to patient level data is possible, or of a decision analytical model, in which access to patient level data may be limited.

Each option for collecting resource use information also has costs and benefits, with patient files and administrative databases sometimes being more complete with the potential to provide a longer time period of retrospective data for the patient. This might be particularly useful for situations where the economic evaluation was not included as part of the original trial design or where a before-and-after design is being used.

Despite this positive feature, patient files may require more resources to collect the information and both sources may have patient consent and confidentiality issues associated with accessing the information.

As databases are usually designed for different purposes than research, they may not have all of the information required or be in a useful format and the interpretation of missing data can be a challenge. For instance the absence of a test in patient notes may be due to the fact that the test did not actually occur or it was just not recorded.

As discussed in §1.3.1, the types of cost and resource data collected depend on the perspective of the decision-maker. For more restricted questions, e.g. looking at the cost of options for a local care pathway, cost information from local financial information (LFI) systems may be sufficient.

LFI is also likely to be more detailed and can be broken down into *fixed* (i.e. not depending on the quantity purchased) and *variable* costs and the relative contributions of staff, consumables, capital and overheads to the total cost of an option. Thus, it can be particularly useful for assessing the cost of a new treatment where other data are not available.

On the other hand, to assess the cost-effectiveness of an option at the national level, sometimes it is expected that broader types of financial information be used. As the cost for a particular treatment or procedure can vary both within and between hospitals, some form of national reference data might be expected to be used to represent the average national cost or reimbursed figure for a given procedure based on diagnosis.

For a number of countries, published data are available in the form of case-mix or reference cost information based on diagnostic related groups (DRGs) or health care related groups. More detailed information on the collection of cost data is available in *Oxford Handbook* texts such as Glick et al. (2007).

1.4 Outcomes

As outlined earlier and, more in detail in §1.6, economic evaluations are the comparison of alternative options not just in terms of their costs but also their consequences. Even if an option has a lower unit cost, it may be the case that more health could be purchased for the same resources if another option were chosen.

For example, Table 1.1 shows the comparison of three hypothetical different options in terms of the unit cost and the total health that can be purchased with a fixed monetary unit (say, for definiteness, 100).

Although option A is the cheapest per unit, if a decision-maker has 100 monetary units, by purchasing 20 units of A the total health benefit forgone if the same resources were used to purchase B is $(15 - 12) = 3$ health units. Similarly, if they purchased C, the total health benefit lost would be $(16.25 - 12) = 4.25$ health units. If cost and outcome information are not combined in some principled way, then there is inadequate information available to the decision-maker to decide which option to choose in order to achieve the greatest health benefit within finite resources.

TABLE 1.1
Comparison across 3 hypothetical options of total health purchased with 100 monetary units

Option	Cost per unit	Health outcomes per unit	Units purchased per 100	Total health purchased
A	5	0.6	20.00	12.00
B	10	1.5	10.00	15.00
C	8	1.3	12.50	16.25

For some analyses within a specific clinical area, "hard" clinical outcomes can be used in the economic evaluations. These will usually take the form of the outcome of the programme of most interest, e.g. cases of tuberculosis (TB) prevented for a TB screening programme (Pareek et al., 2011), days of normal functioning gained for patients with schizophrenia that have received cognitive behavioural therapy (van der Gaag et al., 2011), or life years saved as part of a colorectal cancer screening programme (van Rossum et al., 2011). When combined with the associated costs, these types of analysis can be particularly useful for decision-makers working with budget limitations for a particular disease area (Drummond et al., 2005).

However, these analyses are affected by problems such as the difficulty in comparing across disease areas unless the same outcome is used (e.g. life years saved). Moreover, they might miss out important information related to morbidity or disease progression that is not captured by summary statistics.

Despite these possible limitations, hard clinical outcomes are also important for decision analytical models. Clinical outcomes such as the proportion of patients that suffer a specific clinical episode (e.g. a relapse; movement through different stages of a disease such as disease progression in cancer; and mortality rates) can be used to calculate values in the model. These might then be translated in *transition probabilities* that can be used in evaluations based on Markov models (cfr. §5.4).

1.4.1   Condition specific outcomes

Condition specific outcome measures are those that are designed to pick up the changes in health outcomes specific to a disease. This can be through descriptions of different levels of a disease, vignettes or standardised condition specific measures (Brazier et al., 2007b).

Different instruments have been put together with the aim of creating a practical, open-access database of resource-use questionnaires for use by trial health economists and can be accessed from http://www.dirum.org.

1.4.2   Generic outcomes

The argument for generic instruments for measuring health outcomes is that, because they have a standardised description of health, they allow for a comparison of outcomes across different disease areas and hence are preferred by decision-making bodies (NICE, 2008).

The strength of condition specific measures, i.e. that they measure characteristics most pertinent to a disease, is also a weakness in that they are usually less broad than generic measures. Therefore, they do not measure wider contributors to health and well-being or capture information on co-morbidities (Brazier et al., 2007a).

General health profiles such as the *Short Form 36* (SF-36), the *Nottingham Health Profile* and the *Sickness Impact Profile* provide a comprehensive overview of health and well-being, but are less useful in economic evaluations as they do not provide a single index score to allow for easy comparisons across different economic evaluations (Drummond et al., 2005).

The preferred measures for economic evaluations are short health questionnaires that measure patients' health and well-being across a number of domains, such as pain, mobility, depression and usual activities. This information is then converted into a single utility index using a standardised algorithm. The main examples are the *EuroQol 5D* (EQ-5D, http://www.euroqol.org) and the *Short Form 6 Dimension* (SF-6D, http://www.shef.ac.uk/scharr/sections/heds/mvh/sf-6d), which is shortened version of the SF-36.

The EQ-5D questionnaire

The EQ-5D (Kind et al., 2005) is a short questionnaire primarily designed for self-completion by respondents. Thus, it is particularly effective when used in postal surveys, clinics or face-to-face interviews. The questionnaire consists of two parts: the first one, shown in Figure 1.3, is a descriptive system about the health dimensions considered as most relevant. These are *mobility, self-care, usual activities, pain/discomfort* and *anxiety/depression.* In the most recent version, each dimension has 5 levels: "no problems," "slight problems," "moderate problems," "severe problems" and "extreme problems," and respondents are asked to indicate their health state by ticking in the box against the most appropriate statement.

Under each heading, please tick ONE box that best describes your health TODAY

MOBILITY
I have no problems in walking about ☐
I have slight problems in walking about ☐
I have moderate problems in walking about ☐
I have severe problems in walking about ☐
I am unable to walk about ☐

SELF-CARE
I have no problems washing or dressing myself ☐
I have slight problems washing or dressing myself ☐
I have moderate problems washing or dressing myself ☐
I have severe problems washing or dressing myself ☐
I am unable to wash or dress myself ☐

USUAL ACTIVITIES (e.g. work, study, housework, family or leisure activities)
I have no problems doing my usual activities ☐
I have slight problems doing my usual activities ☐
I have moderate problems doing my usual activities ☐
I have severe problems doing my usual activities ☐
I am unable to do my usual activities ☐

PAIN / DISCOMFORT
I have no pain or discomfort ☐
I have slight pain or discomfort ☐
I have moderate pain or discomfort ☐
I have severe pain or discomfort ☐
I have extreme pain or discomfort ☐

ANXIETY / DEPRESSION
I am not anxious or depressed ☐
I am slightly anxious or depressed ☐
I am moderately anxious or depressed ☐
I am severely anxious or depressed ☐
I am extremely anxious or depressed ☐

FIGURE 1.3
The descriptive part of the EQ-5D questionnaire. Source: http://www.euroqol.org

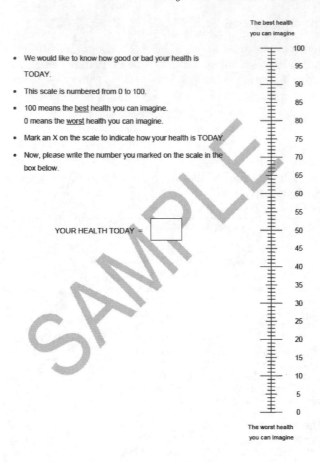

FIGURE 1.4
The visual analogue scale of the EQ-5D questionnaire. Individuals are required to specify their current level of health by selecting a value in the scale from 0 (worst imaginable health) to 100 (best imaginable health). Source: http://www.euroqol.org

In addition, in the second part of the questionnaire respondents are also asked to self-rate their health on a vertical, visual analogue scale where the endpoints are labelled "best imaginable health state" (associated with a score of 100) and "worst imaginable health state" (a score of 0). This information can be used as a quantitative measure of health outcome as judged by the individual respondents. Figure 1.4 shows a sample version of the visual analogue scale. □

The SF-6D measure of health

Unlike the EQ-5D, rather than a proper questionnaire, the SF-6D is a derived generic measure of health, composed of six multi-level dimensions: *physical functioning, role limitation, social functioning, bodily pain, mental health* and *vitality*. The SF-6D is constructed from a sample of 11 items selected from the SF-36 to minimise the loss of descriptive information (Brazier et al., 2002). Thus, if an individual has compiled the SF-36 questionnaire, it is possible to derive the resulting measure of health, as measured by the SF-6D, in a semi-automatic way.

Figure 1.5 shows an excerpt from the SF-36 questionnaire. The responses to the original questions are combined following a pre-specified algorithm to produce a level for each dimension (there are between four and six levels). For example, an individual who responds "Yes, limited a lot" to questions 3a. and 3b. and "Yes, limited a little" to question 3j. is associated with a level of 2 for the physical functioning dimension.

For each dimension, level 1 represents no loss of health or functioning; thus, state 111111 denotes perfect health. On the other hand, the highest value for a given dimension represents the worst possible level of health. Thus the worst possible state (excluding death) is 645655. □

As suggested above, both generic and condition specific measures have strengths and weaknesses for use in economic evaluations. Decision making bodies tend to prefer the use of a generic outcome which has been valued by members of the general population to allow for like-with-like comparisons across disease areas.

However, for conditions where there is legitimate concern regarding the use of a generic measure — e.g. some mental health conditions (Brazier, 2010), chronic fatigue (Brazier et al., 2007b) and urinary tract problems (Brazier et al., 2007a) — or when there is no generic data available, the use of a condition specific measure in an economic evaluation may be accepted by decision-making bodies (NICE, 2008), provided that the condition specific measure be converted to a utility index using direct valuation or mapping, as described below.

1.4.3 Valuing outcomes

Each health state in generic instruments such as the EQ-5D and the SF-6D can be converted into a utility score, where a utility score $u = 1$ represents perfect health and a value of $u = 0$ represents death.

For instance, for the EQ-5D, the utility score is defined between $-\infty$ and 1, and negative values are states considered worse than death. The health state represented by a response of "no problems" for all 5 domains is 1. For a response where the person has "some problems" with self-care but "no-problems" with all other domains the utility is 0.815 (equivalent to a health decrement of 0.185

RAND 36-Item Health Survey 1.0 Questionnaire Items

1. In general, would you say your health is:

Excellent	Very good	Good	Fair	Poor
☐	☐	☐	☐	☐

2. Compared to one year ago, how would you rate your health in general now?

Much better now than a year ago	Somewhat better now than a year ago	About the same as one year ago	Somewhat worse now than one year ago	Much worse now than one year ago
☐	☐	☐	☐	☐

3. The following items are about activities you might do during a typical day. Does your health now limit you in these activities? If so, how much?

	Yes, limited a lot	Yes, limited a little	No, not limited at all
a. Vigorous activities, such as running, lifting heavy objects, participating in strenuous sports	☐	☐	☐
b. Moderate activities, such as moving a table, pushing a vacuum cleaner, bowling, or playing golf?	☐	☐	☐
c. Lifting or carrying groceries	☐	☐	☐
d. Climbing several flights of stairs	☐	☐	☐
e. Climbing one flight of stairs	☐	☐	☐
f. Bending, kneeling or stooping	☐	☐	☐
g. Walking more than one mile	☐	☐	☐
h. Walking several blocks	☐	☐	☐
i. Walking one bloc	☐	☐	☐
j. Bathing or dressing yourself	☐	☐	☐

FIGURE 1.5
An excerpt of the SF-36 questionnaire. Selected items are used to derive the SF-6D measure. Adapted from: www.rand.org/health/surveys_tools/mos/mos_core_36item_survey.html

with respect to perfect health) and for a response where a patient has "extreme problems" for the domains mobility, usual activity, pain and discomfort and "some problems" for the domains self-care and depression/anxiety the utility would be a negative score of −0.319 (indicating that such a state would be perceived as worse than death).

These utility values are computed from members of the general public in the UK using the *time-trade off* (TTO) methodology (Dolan et al., 1995). In TTO, respondents are asked hypothetical situations that trade *quality* for *quantity* of life. Respondents are given a choice between two health states — a health state less than full health for a certain number of years and full health for fewer years. The number of years in full health is varied until respondents are indifferent between the two options (Rowen and Brazier, 2011).

As for the SF-6D, a different approach is used to compute the utility scores, based on the *standard-gamble* (SG) technique. In a SG, the extreme states $y^{\min}$ (e.g. death) and $y^{\max}$ (e.g. perfect health) are identified and arbitrarily associated with a utility score of 0 and 1 respectively. A comparative value for any other health state $y \neq y^{\min}, y^{\max}$ is then obtained by considering the two alternative scenarios:

1. obtain the outcome y (e.g. living for a fixed amount of time in a less-than-perfect health state) with probability 1;

2. obtain the preferred outcome $y^{\max}$ with a given probability π and the worst outcome $y^{\min}$ with probability $(1 - \pi)$.

Respondents are asked to vary the levels of the probability π until they deem the two scenarios as indifferent. The selected level of probability π is then associated as the utility score to the less-than-perfect state.

Larger utilities imply that the respondent would consider a certain event to be equivalent to the uncertain situation in which there is a very high probability of obtaining the preferred outcome. Thus, to exchange a certain situation that is considered to be "good," the respondent needs to be nearly certain of improving the outcome (i.e. get the best possible). Conversely, if an outcome is associated with a small utility, then it only takes a small chance of obtaining the preferred consequence for the respondent to be willing to trade it.

A sample of 249 of the possible health states defined in the SF-6D, selected to ensure a balance of mild, moderate and severe states have been valued by 611 members of the general public in the UK, resulting in 3518 observed SG valuations (Brazier et al., 2002). Suitable statistical models (using both a parametric ordinal regression and a more robust non parametric alternative) have been estimated to predict all the health states described by the SF-6D. Table 1.2 shows some of the results. For example, individuals providing answers to the SF-36 positioning them in levels 321222 for the 6 dimensions of the SF-6D are associated with a utility score of 0.7133.

Unlike TTO, SG satisfies the proposed theory of utility of von Neumann and Morgenstein (1953), because it includes a measure of risk. Nevertheless, as mentioned previously both are called "utility scores" by convention (Drummond et al., 2005). More correctly, both instruments and their associated utility algorithms are called *preference-based* measures of health related quality of life (HRQL), as they include information about the value that people attach to one health state compared to another (McIntosh et al., 2010).

Utility scores are sensitive to the method used to arrive at them, as the different methods use risk and uncertainty differently to determine the value for a health state (Drummond et al., 2005). Whether or not the instrument has

TABLE 1.2

Observed and estimated utility values for selected states. State 111111 denotes perfect health, while state 645655 indicate the worst possible. Adapted from: Karroubi et al. (2007)

Health state	Observed mean	Estimated utility			
		Non parametric		Parametric	
		Mean	*SD*	*Mean*	*SD*
111111	0.9896	1	0	1	0
111112	0.8959	0.9419	0.0284	0.9689	0.0139
111122[a]	—	0.9107	0.0372	0.9333	0.0188
121112	0.6769	0.8175	0.0299	0.9183	0.0176
...	...	...	...	...	...
321222[a]	—	0.7133	0.034	0.8072	0.0244
...	...	...	...	...	...
433433	0.7218	0.6045	0.0326	0.6542	0.0230
...	...	...	...	...	...
645655	0.2130	0.2031	0.0231	0.2582	0.0129

[a] State not observed in the sample

been valued by patients or members of the general public can also influence the utility values for health states (Brazier et al., 2004).

As a result, particularly when synthesising information for a decision analytical model, it is important to note which instrument was used to determine patients' health states in an economic evaluation, which utility algorithm was used and the impact that can have on the results of the analysis.

In cases where a generic measure has been shown to be unresponsive to changes in a disease, a condition specific measure can be used (NICE, 2008). This measure should then be valued using the same methodology as that used to value the standard generic measure for that decision-making body.

In the case of NICE, this requires that the condition specific measure is valued using TTO and by members of the general public (NICE, 2008). An example of a condition specific measure valued for use in economic evaluations includes the *McSad utility score*, a condition specific measure specifically developed to measure depression health states (Bennet et al., 2000).

Another option for attaching utility weights to a condition specific measure is *mapping*. This is possible when patients have completed a generic preference-based measure of HRQL (e.g. the EQ-5D) and a condition specific measure. Statistical techniques such as ordinary least squares or logistic regression can then be used to predict utilities from condition specific responses.

It should be noted that there are some limitations associated with these methodologies and measures of uncertainty in the resulting inferences, e.g. standard errors for the mapping algorithm, should be included in some form of sensitivity analysis (Mortimer and Segal, 2007; Petrillo and Cairns, 2008).

1.5 Discounting

The costs and outcomes of an option can occur at different times in relation to when the actual intervention is implemented. A large body of research suggests that people value benefits that arrive closer to the present time more than they value benefits that they receive later in the future.

Discounting takes into account the differential timing of outcomes and time relative preference by reducing the value of costs and effects seen in the future compared to those seen at present. Thus, it is widely recognised that in any economic evaluation with a time horizon greater than 1 year, costs and outcomes should be discounted by a factor of $(1+d)^j$, where d is the discount rate and j is the time at which the cost or outcomes occur (Drummond et al., 2005).

The discount rate suggested by NICE is 3.5% for all costs and outcomes, although there are differing views about whether this is reasonable and whether costs and outcomes should have a different discount rate (Brouwer et al., 2005). As a result, it is best practice to conduct a sensitivity analysis (cfr. §3.3.4) with discount rates between 0% and 6%.

In general, it is interesting to report the *Present Value* (PV) of an intervention t to quantify its current worth. For example, the PV for the cost of intervention t is computed as

$$\mathrm{PV}_t^{(c)} = \sum_{j=0}^{J} \frac{c_{tj}}{(1+d)^j}, \tag{1.1}$$

where c_{tj} is the cost associated with intervention t at time j and J is the number of time points selected for the analysis. Similar reasoning can be followed to derive the present value in terms of the clinical outcome measure chosen for a given intervention.

Example: computing the present value

Suppose that a given health intervention used to control an infective disease is analysed. The annual direct cost of implementation is £15 000 and the programme has a time horizon of five years, including the present one. Assuming that a discount rate of 3.5% (i.e. 0.035) is used, the present value of the programme is:

$$
\begin{aligned}
\text{PV} &= \frac{£15\,000}{(1+0.035)^0} + \frac{£15\,000}{(1+0.035)^1} + \frac{£15\,000}{(1+0.035)^2} + \\
&\quad \frac{£15\,000}{(1+0.035)^3} + \frac{£15\,000}{(1+0.035)^4} \\
&= £15\,000.00 + £14\,492.75 + £14\,002.66 + \\
&\quad £13\,529.14 + £13\,071.63 \\
&= £70\,096.19.
\end{aligned}
$$

The present value is different (in fact is less) than the value that would be obtained by multiplying the annual cost by the number of years considered (i.e. $£15\,000 \times 5 = £75\,000$), just because this quantity is given a different weight at each different time point. □

1.6 Types of economic evaluations

There are at least three major types of economic evaluations that are formally applied to health economic problems: cost-benefit analysis, cost-effectiveness analysis and cost-utility analysis, which we review in some detail below. An additional methodology is represented by cost-minimisation analysis, but as it is rarely used we will only describe it briefly.

1.6.1 Cost-minimisation analysis

Cost-minimisation analysis (CMA) is arguably the simplest form of economic evaluation. In a CMA, the benefits of two or more options have been established as equivalent and therefore the focus is exclusively on a comparison of the costs associated with each.

CMA is rarely used in practice, because there are limited instances where the benefits of two or more options are indeed equivalent. Moreover, as CMA requires that equivalence is already established prior to data collection, it is not a viable analysis option for clinical trials.

In addition, CMA has also been criticised because, in only considering costs, it does not allow for the investigation of uncertainty surrounding the benefits (Briggs and O' Brien, 2001), which is an important component of economic evaluations, as will be explored further in §3.4.

As a result of its limited scope, CMA will not be discussed further in this book.

1.6.2   Cost-benefit analysis

Cost-benefit analysis (CBA) requires that all costs and benefits of each option being investigated are calculated, converted into the same units and added up to provide a total figure for that option. The common units used are usually monetary (e.g. Pound, Euro, Dollar or Yen[1]).

Different options can be compared based on the total final figure, with the option that delivers the most benefits compared to the associated cost (i.e. the option with the largest value), usually deemed as the best alternative. Consequently, CBA results in a single monetary value for each option, making it easy for the decision-maker to compare a number of different interventions. This characteristic is often considered as its main strength.

Nevertheless, CBA presents challenges for economic evaluations in health care due to the ethical and logistical difficulties associated with valuing the outcomes of health care in monetary units. For instance, CBA assumes that a monetary value can be given to quantities that do not logically relate to money; e.g. the monetary value associated with changes in blood pressure.

People can also feel uncomfortable valuing in monetary terms quantities that have a strong relationship with basic human rights such as disability- or mental illness-free or extra years of life. In addition, some outcomes of health care are also hard to measure, e.g. how a patient feels about being more independent as a result of reduced disability.

Although some economic evaluations include components of CBA, in the sense that all the quantities in the analysis are converted to a monetary unit, the scope of most economic evaluations in health care is rarely wide enough to be considered a true CBA.

This is because, typically, such analyses do not include an assessment of *all* costs and benefits; sometimes they only include the costs and benefits from a specific perspective (cfr. §1.3.1) and most will only include an analysis of a single health outcome of interest, usually a generic outcome which allows for comparisons across disease areas (cfr. §1.6.4).

Nevertheless, CBAs are becoming more popular, particularly in public health economic evaluations, due to the inclusion of all costs and benefits across different sectors and the ability to consider a wider range of health impacts. For instance, an evaluation of a tax on older cars can include factors such as: *i)* the extra revenue to the government associated with the tax; *ii)* a monetary valuation of improved air quality and environmental improvements from reduced pollution from those who sell their cars to avoid the tax; *iii)* the savings associated with reduced hospital use due to reductions in respiratory related hospital admissions; and *iv)* the impact on the economy of new cars being bought to replace the old ones.

There is also ongoing research to address some of the problems outlined

---

[1]Most of the examples discussed in this book are related with the British context and therefore we usually consider Pounds (£) as the monetary unit of interest. However, all our arguments, models and computations apply directly to any currency.

above with using CBA to evaluate health care. The measurement of patient outcomes has been progressing in the health care field with increased interest in development and testing of a wide range of patient reported outcome measures (PROMs) that determine and measure the attributes most important to patients (Dawson et al., 2010). There is also an increasing volume of literature regarding the willingness-to-pay for different health outcomes (McIntosh et al., 2010). The combination of this work represents a better way to capture and value the consequences of health care from a patient perspective.

An example of CBA

Consider an analysis of the implementation of a hypothetical vaccination strategy to prevent some infectious disease, particularly relevant to young children. Vaccination for the disease can be made available to *a)* children attending primary school (which we indicate as $t = 1$); or *b)* children attending both primary and secondary school ($t = 2$).

Suppose further that the vaccine is perfectly effective, i.e. when a child is vaccinated the occurrence of the disease will be prevented. Conversely, when a child becomes ill with the disease, the standard course of treatment consists in hospitalisation for a week. This is clearly an unrealistic scenario in real practice, but we adopt it here to avoid unnecessary complications in discussing the main points of CBA.

Estimations of incidence rates of the disease (ρ_1 and ρ_2 respectively for children in primary and secondary schools) and about the costs of administration and acquisition of the vaccine (v), as well as hospitalisation (h) are presented in Table 1.3, together with the sample sizes for the two sub-groups (indicated by N_1 and N_2).

TABLE 1.3
Estimation for costs, incidence rates and reference population for the hypothetical vaccination problem

Cost measures	
Vaccination cost (acquisition + administration, v)	£12
Hospitalisation (1 week, h)	£700
Disease incidence rate	
Primary school (ρ_1)	0.1427
Secondary school (ρ_2)	0.0548
Reference populations (sample sizes)	
Primary school (N_1)	4 093 710
Secondary school (N_2)	3 252 140

Using the available data, it is possible to compute the overall cost associated with the two strategies:

$$\begin{aligned} c_1 &= v \times N_1 \\ &= \pounds 12 \times 4\,093\,710 = \pounds 49\,124\,520 \end{aligned}$$

and

$$\begin{aligned} c_2 &= v \times (N_1 + N_2) \\ &= \pounds 12 \times (4\,093\,710 + 3\,252\,140) = \pounds 88\,150\,200. \end{aligned}$$

As for the benefits, we consider the gain deriving from the vaccination strategies expressed in terms of cost averted for the hospitalisation events (and thus the higher, the better). Then we can compute:

$$\begin{aligned} b_1 &= h \times \rho_1 \times N_1 \\ &= \pounds 700 \times 0.1427 \times 4\,093\,710 = \pounds 408\,920\,692, \end{aligned}$$

for the strategy that makes the vaccine available only to children in primary school and

$$\begin{aligned} b_2 &= h \times [(\rho_1 \times N_1) + (\rho_2 \times N_2)] \\ &= \pounds 700 \times (584\,172.4 + 178\,217.3) = \pounds 533\,672\,790, \end{aligned}$$

for the alternative strategy where both primary and secondary schools have access to it.

Consequently, the cost-benefit ratios (CBR) for the two options are:

$$\text{CBR}_1 = \frac{c_1}{b_1} = \frac{\pounds 49\,124\,520}{\pounds 408\,920\,692} = 0.1201$$

and

$$\text{CBR}_2 = \frac{c_2}{b_2} = \frac{\pounds 88\,150\,200}{\pounds 533\,672\,790} = 0.1652.$$

Since $\text{CBR}_2 > \text{CBR}_1$, the favourite option is *b)*. In fact, despite having a cost that is nearly double that of strategy *a)*, vaccinating both primary and secondary school children produces a health benefit that outweighs the extra costs.

Because both the numerator and the denominator of the cost-benefit ratio are expressed in monetary units, this quantity is a pure number. Therefore, it is possible to directly compare the CBRs of two different comparisons (e.g. $t = 1$ versus $t = 0$ and $t = 3$ versus $t = 2$). □

1.6.3   Cost-effectiveness analysis

As mentioned above, CBA can be less suitable for economic evaluations in health care because of the problems associated with valuing health related outcomes. This can be overcome using a cost-effectiveness analysis (CEA) instead. A CEA can be broadly described as an evaluation of the *cost-per-outcome gained* (cfr. §1.7 for more details).

Usually, the outcome considered in a CEA is a familiar and clinically relevant measurement, e.g. blood pressure test scores or mortality rates. Consequently, CEA is often preferred as an economic evaluation method by health care professionals and other health care stakeholders, since it avoids impinging any monetary value judgement on the outcome.

On the other hand, because the health outcome has no direct monetary value, in situations where an option costs more and results in better outcomes compared to another option, it is hard to assess if the gains are worth the additional resources required. In economic term, this is known as the *opportunity cost* (cfr. §3.5.2), i.e. the cost associated with the fact that resources allocated to a particular option are not available for other treatment options that could have resulted in better outcomes.

The limited resources in health care mean that decision-makers might need to make a decision about where to remove resources from, in order to pay for the new treatment. Unfortunately, the use of disease-specific outcomes in cost-effectiveness analyses means that comparisons across different analyses and disease might be difficult to make.

For example, suppose that an analysis finds that treatment $t = 1$ results in 5 units decrease on blood pressure for every 1 000 monetary units spent in comparison to *treatment as usual* (generally indicated as $t = 0$); similarly, treatment $t = 2$ results in 3 less days of heavy drinking per month for every 1 000 monetary units spent compared to $t = 0$. From the decision-maker point of view, it is hard to decide which combination of $t = 1, 2$ would result in the best outcomes *for the overall population*, given that, for every unit of $t = 2$ purchased, forgoes the ability to purchase some of $t = 1$.

Another problem of cost-effectiveness analyses is that, because they do not use natural units, it can be hard to assess more than one benefit from a treatment: there is no way to combine information about a treatment that reduces high blood pressure and also results in gains in years of life lived as their units are not naturally additive or multiplicative.

1.6.4   Cost-utility analysis

To overcome the problems associated with CEA, health care decision-makers tend to prefer the use of a common health outcome unit, so that comparable decisions can be made across different disease areas.

A cost-utility analysis (CUA) can still be summarised as an incremental cost per unit change in outcome, much as CEA. However, in a CUA, the outcome combines information about morbidity, or quality of life, and mortality to arrive at a *quality-adjusted life year* (QALY, Loomes and McKenzie, 1989).

The basic idea of QALYs is quite intuitive: life expectancy of one year of perfect health is associated with a value of 1, while death is associated with a value of 0. Other possible health states are ranked between these two extremes, although sometimes negative values for states worse than death are also possible — some conceptual problems with states worse than death have been noted and mechanisms to handle them explored, for instance by Devlin et al. (2011). Operationally, QALYs are calculated by multiplying the amount of time spent in a given health state by the preference-based value (i.e. the *utility*) attached to that health state (cfr. §1.4.3).

Because of its wide popularity in the field of health economic evaluation, CUA is often intended as a generalised term for all cost-per-QALY analyses, and hence it can refer to a broad range of methodologies, each of which can have different results. Thus, some caution is suggested in comparing findings.

In the rest of the book, we refer to CEA and CUA almost interchangeably; the analytical methods developed in Chapter 3 are indeed applicable to both, provided the correct definition of the outcome measure is used.

Example: computing QALYs

Table 1.4 shows a hypothetical example of utility scores, QALYs and costs for a patient in a treatment group compared to a patient in a control group, over a period of 2 years.

At baseline (i.e. time 0), both patients are assumed to have the same utility, $u_{t0} = 0.656$ (here $t = 0$ indicates the control, while $t = 1$ is the active treatment group). For each patient, we also assume four extra measurements u_{tj}, for $j = 1, 2, 3, 4$ at 6, 12, 18 and 24 months, respectively. As is clear from Table 1.4, for $j = 1, 2, 3$, u_{1j} is consistently higher than u_{0j}, while $u_{04} = u_{14} = 0.744$. For example, these utility scores might have been computed starting from health questionnaires or health measures, such as the EQ-5D or the SF-6D.

In addition, the cost associated with each treatment and each time points are also recorded as c_{tj}. In the active intervention group, there is a higher entry cost (perhaps due to the acquisition of the technology), while the remaining time periods are associated with the same amount of £300.

To compute the QALYs between two consecutive measurements $(j - 1)$ and j, we simply compute the average of the two utility scores and rescale the time period between the two measurements, with respect to the reference time, which is defined as one year:

$$q_{tj} = \frac{\left(u_{t(j-1)} + u_{tj}\right)}{2} \delta_j$$

where

$$\delta_j = \frac{\text{time between measurements } j \text{ and } (j - 1), \text{ in years}}{1 \text{ year}}$$

TABLE 1.4

An example of calculation of QALYs from utility scores. In the two treatment groups $(t = 0, 1)$, the measurements consist of the utility score u_{tj} and the costs c_{tj}, for $j = 0, \ldots, 4$ occasions

	Baseline	6 months	12 months	18 months	24 months	Total
Treatment group $(t = 1)$						
Utility score	0.656	0.744	0.85	0.744	0.744	
QALYs		0.350	0.399	0.399	0.372	1.519
Costs		£2 300	£300	£300	£300	£3 200
Control group $(t = 0)$						
Utility score	0.656	0.656	0.656	0.656	0.744	
QALYs		0.328	0.328	0.328	0.350	1.334
Costs		£300	£300	£300	£300	£1 200
Difference						
in QALYs $(\mathrm{E}[\Delta_e])^a$						0.185
in costs $(\mathrm{E}[\Delta_c])^a$						£2 000
Cost per QALY^a						£10 811

^{a} These quantities are defined in §1.7

For example, the QALYs at 6 months (i.e. at time $j = 1$) for treatment $t = 0$ are computed as

$$q_{01} = \left(\frac{0.656 + 0.656}{2}\right)\left(\frac{0.5}{1}\right) = 0.164,$$

since the time between the two measurements, 6 months, is only half a year. Similarly, for $t = 1$ the computation gives

$$q_{11} = \left(\frac{0.656 + 0.744}{2}\right)\left(\frac{0.5}{1}\right) = 0.35.$$

Overall, for each treatment the QALYs can be computed by summing the q_{tj} terms across all the time periods. In the present example, the measurements are repeated at 6 month intervals and thus all values are added up over the 2 years. We define the QALYs using the notation e_t (to indicate the "effectiveness" of the treatment) as

$$e_t = \sum_{j=1}^{J} q_{tj}.$$

This produces a result of 1.519 extra QALYs for the patient under $t = 1$ and only 1.334 extra QALYs for the single patient under $t = 0$.

Notice that, in more realistic cases, instead of a single patient per group, we would have access to a sample of patients and therefore the relevant measures would be the population average computed across all relevant individuals. □

Each of the three main types of economic evaluation described above has strengths and weaknesses, and although each has its own specific characteristics most economic evaluations generally combine aspects of each. More in depth information can be found in Drummond et al. (2005). NICE's Decision Support Unit also has extensive guidance to support technical appraisals http://www.nicedsu.org.uk/. Table 1.5 summarises the main differences among them.

TABLE 1.5

A comparison of the characteristics of the main types of economic evaluation. Adapted from Meltzer and Teutsch (1998)

Type	Costs included[a]		Outcomes
	Direct	*Indirect*	
Cost-benefit	✓	✓	Monetary unit
Cost-effectiveness	✓	often	Health outcome[b]
Cost-utility	✓	rarely	Utility measure[c]

[a] All future costs and benefits should be discounted to the reference year (cfr. §1.5)
[b] For example: number of deaths averted
[c] For example: QALYs (cfr. §1.6.4)

1.7 Comparing health interventions

As discussed earlier, the purpose of economic evaluations is to provide information to decision-makers about the costs and outcomes of health care options to help with resource allocation decisions. Generally, economic summaries are computed in the form of "cost-per-outcome" ratios.

Moreover, in order to compare the two interventions ($t = 0, 1$), we can define suitable incremental population summaries, such as the population average *increment in benefits*, suitably measured as utilities (as in a CUA) or by means of hard clinical outcomes (as in a CEA):

$$\mathrm{E}[\Delta_e] = \bar{e}_1 - \bar{e}_0 \qquad (1.2)$$

and the population average *increment in costs*:

$$\mathrm{E}[\Delta_c] = \bar{c}_1 - \bar{c}_0, \qquad (1.3)$$

where $\bar{e}_t, \bar{c}_t$ are the population averages of suitable measures of benefit and cost, respectively.

These in turn can be used to compute the *Incremental Cost-Effectiveness Ratio* (ICER), defined as

$$\text{ICER} = \frac{\text{E}[\Delta_c]}{\text{E}[\Delta_e]}. \tag{1.4}$$

The ICER represents the cost per incremental unit of effectiveness (e.g. cost per QALY gained, or cost per death/event averted) and it provides a ratio summary of the additional cost and outcomes (also called effects) that result from one option compared to another.

For example, in a CUA the value used in the denominator is a standardised utility index based on general public preferences that allows for comparisons across different disease areas. Outcome information and cost information are combined to provide meaningful information to decisions-makers about each option.

Example: computing the ICER

Consider again the example of Table 1.4. Extending the reasoning followed to compute the QALYs, the overall cost of each treatment group can be computed by summing over the repeated measurements, which leads to an overall cost of $c_1 = £3\,200$ for the patient under $t = 1$ and of $c_0 = £1\,200$ for the patient under $t = 0$. Notice that in this case, in order to simplify matters, we do not consider discounting, although the time horizon considered is 2 years and therefore it would be more appropriate to do so.

As reported in Table 1.4, the increment in costs is $\text{E}[\Delta_c] = £(3\,200 - 1\,200) = £2\,000$, while the increment in QALYs is $\text{E}[\Delta_e] = (1.519 - 1.334) = 0.185$ (recall that in this trivial case, there is only one patient per group and therefore the observed values are identical with the population means). Thus, the ICER (i.e. the cost per QALY) can be computed as the ratio

$$\begin{aligned} \text{ICER} \quad &= \quad \frac{\text{E}[\Delta_c]}{\text{E}[\Delta_e]} \\ &= \quad \frac{£2\,000}{0.185}, \end{aligned}$$

which equals £10 811 per QALYs.   □

Despite having been historically considered as an appropriate measure of economic evaluation, the use of the ICER has been widely criticised because of some major limitations (Spiegelhalter et al., 2004).

For example, knowing the sign of the ICER is not sufficient to identify the optimal treatment: an ICER of £100 can be derived by values of $(\text{E}[\Delta_e], \text{E}[\Delta_c]) = (2, 200)$, indicating that the new treatment produces on average an increase in effectiveness of 2 units at the cost of an extra £200, as well as by the values $(E[\Delta_e], E[\Delta_c]) = (-2, -200)$, a case in which the new intervention is less effective, but cheaper.

Moreover, from the statistical point of view the ICER can have infinite variance and it is generally difficult to perform interval estimation for its values.

1.7.1 The cost-effectiveness plane

To help disentangle the difficulties in the interpretation of the value of the ICER for the comparison between two interventions, it is helpful to consider the graphical representation provided by the *cost-effectiveness plane*. This is a visual description of the incremental costs and effects of an option compared to some standard intervention.

Consider the situation depicted in Figure 1.6. Suppose there are 6 different interventions available; one is considered to be the current standard, while the remaining 5 are used to produce pairwise comparisons with respect to it.

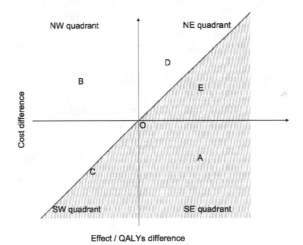

Effect / QALYs difference

FIGURE 1.6
The cost-effectiveness plane for the 5 pairwise comparisons against some reference interventions. The 45° line indicates the decision-maker's *willingness-to-pay*. Options below the line (i.e. those lying in the grey area) are "sustainable," in the sense that the extra cost required is more than offset by the gain in effects.

The point O indicates the origin of the plane, i.e. the point where the differentials of costs and effects are both equal to 0, indicating no difference between the two interventions being compared. We can think of this point as representing the option used as a comparator. Similarly, the resulting ICERs for all the other comparisons are indicated by the letters A, B, C, D and E in Figure 1.6.

Option A in the southeastern quadrant shows a negative cost differential (which means that it cost less than the comparator) and also results in more QALYs. Thus it is referred to as a "dominant" option. It would be the chosen intervention in a CEA.

Option B in the northwestern quadrant costs more and also results in fewer QALYs than O and hence is dominated by the comparator.

Options D, E and C have a much less clear interpretation. Option C costs less but also results in fewer QALYs than O; thus it is unclear whether this option should be adopted.

Options D and E in the northeastern quadrant cost more but also result in more QALYs than O. Options such as D and E represent the most common results of an economic evaluation and require the application of a proper decision rule in order to identify their feasibility.

The diagonal in Figure 1.6 can be considered as a *"willingness-to-pay"* (WTP) threshold, in that all values that fall below that line (e.g. E and A), are acceptable, or sustainable, to adopt in comparison to O. This is because the cost for each additional QALY is less than the value which the decision-maker is willing to pay to acquire an additional QALY.

Option D, on the other hand, is above the WTP threshold, because it costs more than the decision-maker is willing to pay for an additional QALY and therefore, while theoretically preferable to O, it is not sustainable and thus will not be selected.

There is no definitive WTP value for a QALY; rather it is up to the decision-makers to decide what they are willing to pay for an additional unit of benefit gained. Normally used thresholds are in the interval £20 000—£30 000 per QALY gained (NICE, 2008). This is in general considered as a reference value throughout Europe, while no fixed amount of a WTP for a QALY gained is established in the US. Approximations vary widely depending on the methodology used (King et al., 2005).

Other, more sophisticated methods to deal with inconsistencies in the ICER are discussed in §3.3.3.

2

Introduction to Bayesian inference

2.1 Introduction

In the context of statistical problems, the frequentist (or empirical) interpretation of probability has played a predominant role throughout the twentieth century, especially in the medical field. In this approach, probability is defined as the limiting frequency of occurrence in an infinitely repeated experiment.

The underlying assumption is that of a "fixed" concept of probability, which is unknown but can be theoretically disclosed by means of repeated trials, under the same experimental conditions. Moreover, probability is generally regarded in classical statistics as a physical property of the object of the analysis.

However, although the frequentist approach still plays the role of the standard in various applied areas, there are many other possible conceptualisations of probability characterising different philosophies behind the problem of statistical inference. Among these, an increasingly popular one is the Bayesian (sometimes referred to as subjectivist, in its contemporary form), originated by the posthumous work of Reverend Thomas Bayes (1763) and the independent contributions by Pierre Simone Laplace (1774, 1812) — see Howie (2002), Senn (2003), Fienberg (2006) or Bertsch McGrayne (2011) for a historical account of Bayesian statistics.

The main feature of this approach is that probability is interpreted as a subjective degree of belief in the occurrence of an event, representing the individual level of uncertainty in its actual realisation (cfr. de Finetti, 1974, probably the most comprehensive account of subjective probability). One of the main implications of subjectivism is that there is no requirement that one should be able to specify, or even conceive of some relevant sequence of repetitions of the event in question, as happens in the frequentist framework, with the advantage that "one-off" type of events can be assessed consistently (Dawid, 2005).

In the Bayesian philosophy, the probability assigned to any event depends on the individual whose uncertainty is being expressed and on the state of background information in light of which this assessment is being made. As any of these factors changes, so too might the probability. Consequently, under the subjectivist view, there is no assumption of a unique, correct (or "true") value for the probability of any uncertain event. Rather, each individual is entitled to their own subjective probability and according to the evidence that becomes sequentially available, they tend to update their belief.

The development of Bayesian applied research has been limited, probably because of the common perception among practitioners that Bayesian methods are "more complex." In fact, in our opinion the apparent higher degree of complexity is more than compensated by at least the two following consequences. First, Bayesian methods allow taking into account, through a formal and consistent model, all the available information, e.g. the results of previous studies. Moreover, the inferential process is straightforward, as it is possible to make probabilistic statements directly on the quantities of interest (i.e. some unobservable feature of the process under study, typically — but not necessarily — represented by a set of parameters).

In our opinion, Bayesian methods allow the practitioner to make the most of the evidence: in just the situation of "repeated trials," after observing the outcomes (e.g. successes and failures) of many past trials (and no other collateral information), all subjectivists will be drawn to an assessment of the probability of obtaining a success on the next event that is extremely close to the observed proportion of successes so far. However, if past data are not sufficiently extensive, it may reasonably be argued that there should indeed be scope for interpersonal disagreement as to the implications of the evidence. Therefore the Bayesian approach provides a more general framework for the problem of statistical inference.

Justifications for the use of Bayesian methods in health care evaluation have been detailed by Spiegelhalter et al. (2004), in terms of the formal quantitative inclusion of external evidence in all aspects of clinical research, including design, analysis, interpretation and policy-making. In particular, the Bayesian approach is valuable because: *i)* it proves more flexible and capable of adapting to each unique situation; *ii)* it represents a more efficient inferential tool, making use of all available evidence and not restricting formal evaluations to just the current data at hand; *iii)* it is particularly effective in producing predictions and inputs for decision-making.

Jackman (2009) suggests that performing statistical analysis by means of Bayesian methods also produces advantages from a pragmatic point of view: because of the wide availability of fast and cheap computing power, simulation-based procedures have allowed researchers to exploit more and more complex statistical models, especially under the Bayesian paradigm. Examples include the possibility of computing interval estimations in a straightforward way, without the need to rely on asymptotic arguments. This in turn has the potential of rendering "hard statistical problems easier."

The account of Bayesian statistics that is presented in this chapter is far from exhaustive — more comprehensive references are O'Hagan (1994), Berry (1996), Bernardo and Smith (1999), Lindley (2000), Robert (2001), Lee (2004), Spiegelhalter et al. (2004), Gelman et al. (2004), Lindley (2006), Lancaster (2008), Carlin and Louis (2009), Jackman (2009) and Christensen et al. (2011).

2.2 Subjective probability and Bayes theorem

The main characteristic of the Bayesian approach is the fact that uncertainty about the occurrence of some event of interest E is not necessarily a physical property of the event, but rather a relationship between the individual expressing the evaluation of such uncertainty and the event. Thus, each individual is entitled to express a different gradation of the uncertainty about a set of events.

This gradation is usually referred to as *degree of belief* in the occurrence of E. We indicate this intuitively as be(E) and we note that this notation only refers to a *qualitative* evaluation of the degree of uncertainty on the occurrence of E. Obviously, a high degree of belief expresses the fact that the individual does not consider E as very uncertain. The maximum degree of belief is obtained when the event E is certain to obtain; similarly, the minimum degree of belief is when it is certain that E will not happen. These two extreme conditions represent *logical* constraints; however, in almost all practical cases, it is not possible to completely eliminate uncertainty about relevant events.

2.2.1 Probability as a measure of uncertainty against a standard

A reasonable way of measuring *quantitatively* the individual degree of belief in E is to associate each random event with a number $\Pr(E)$, which we use to describe the individual's attitude (for this reason, these are sometimes referred to as *personal* probabilities). In other words, $\Pr(E)$ represents a measure of be(E).

In measurement problems it is useful to identify a standard to be used (at least conceptually) as a reference for practical comparisons. In the case of measurement of uncertainty, the easiest situation is perhaps that of an experiment involving draws with replacement from an urn containing n balls that are perfectly identical with one another, except for their color: r balls are red, while b are black (with $r + b = n$).

If the assumption that the balls are indistinguishable (apart from the color) holds, then the degree of belief in the event $R = $ "*draw a red ball*" is intuitively quantifiable as the proportion of red balls in the urn, i.e. $\Pr(R) := r/n$. This definition (often referred to as "classical") can be extended as a reference model to identify the uncertainty about a generic event E.

Consider for instance the event $S = $ "*U. C. Sampdoria will win the next Italian football league.*" This is obviously an uncertain event, since it will obtain (or not) in the future. We are interested in finding a measure of the uncertainty about S, $\Pr(S)$.

In order to do so, we can conceive, at least theoretically, of another uncertain event R representing the selection of a red ball from an urn containing n balls, of which an unspecified number r are red. We consider R as a standard against which we compare our uncertainty on S, to produce the evaluation required.

In particular, if we assumed $r = 0$, this would effectively mean that our degree of belief in S is higher than that in R. This is because in this case R would be logically impossible, since $\Pr(R) = 0/n = 0$. Similarly, if we fixed $r = n$, in comparison our degree of belief in S would be lower than that in R, which in this case would be certain to obtain: $\Pr(R) = n/n = 1$ (notice that we assume that S is an uncertain event, so its probability cannot be 0 or 1).

An increasingly higher degree of belief in R corresponds to increasing the number r in the interval $[0, n]$ of red balls in the urn; formally, the degree of belief in R is strictly monotonically increasing. Moreover, since for $r = 0$: $\mathrm{be}(R) < \mathrm{be}(S)$, but for $r = n$: $\mathrm{be}(R) > \mathrm{be}(S)$, there will exist an intermediate degree r^* for which $\mathrm{be}(R) \equiv \mathrm{be}(S)$.

In fact, the number r^* is unique: if two such values existed $r' \neq r''$ so that for $r = r'$: $\mathrm{be}(R) \equiv \mathrm{be}(S)$ and for $r = r''$: $\mathrm{be}(R) \equiv \mathrm{be}(S)$, then for both these values of r we would have the same degree of belief in R, which is not possible since $\mathrm{be}(R)$ is strictly monotonically increasing with the number of red balls in the urn.

Consequently, it is possible to measure the uncertainty on a given event E in terms of the subjective probability $\Pr(E)$, defined as the proportion r/n of red balls in an urn for which the event R, representing the random selection of a red ball, is associated with the same uncertainty that is currently present on E. In other words, the subjectivist procedure measures uncertainty on a given event by comparison to a standard model. This is done by adjusting the number of red balls in the urn until the value for which the degree of belief in E is *perceived*, or *judged* to be the same as that in R.

Notice that the classical definition is simply instrumental to the formalisation of subjective probability. In fact, there is no reason why the event S needs to be associated with a probability computed as the ratio of the number of "favourable" cases (1, i.e. Sampdoria actually wins the league) to the number of "possible" cases (20, the total number of teams participating in the league). However, using a very simple construction (such as that represented by the urn model) allows, at least conceptually, to identify a universal measure of uncertainty.

In a similar way, there is no logical reason why this evaluation needs to be constant for each individual; for instance, for a person who has no knowledge whatsoever about the Italian football league, $\Pr(S) = 1/20$ might represent a reasonable measure of uncertainty. On the other hand, somebody with extensive expertise in this matter might provide a different value, as a function of the strength they assign to that team.

This highlights the fact that probability is effectively *conditional* on the state of relevant knowledge, which we indicate with $\mathcal{D}$ (background data), available to the individual making the assessment. Thus, a more informative notation to express the degree of belief in a random event, and given the background information is $\Pr(E \mid \mathcal{D})$ — cfr. Dawid (1979) for a technical discussion of conditional probabilities.

Finally, it is important to notice that, unlike in the frequentist approach, the concept of *repetition* of the event E is not important at all in the Bayesian definition of probability. In the standard measurement (and therefore *a fortiori* in the subjective assessment), the long-run frequency with which red or black balls are selected in repeated drawings is irrelevant. To a Bayesian, the relative frequency with which an event occurs is just a quantity that *can* (but does not have to) be used to estimate $\Pr(E)$.

2.2.2   Fundamental rules of probability

While the above definition of subjective probability is conceptually reasonable, to compare a single event to the standard urn model is not operationally viable for most real situations[1]. However, by using this simple model it is possible to derive a set of fundamental rules that generate a methodology capable of helping an individual in a *rational* quantification of their uncertainty. We briefly review them, following closely the argument shown in Lindley (2006).

Convexity: For each event E and conditionally on the background information $\mathcal{D}$, $\Pr(E \mid \mathcal{D})$ is a number between 0 and 1. If, given $\mathcal{D}$, E is known without uncertainty, then its probability is 1.

Additivity: For each pair of events E, F and conditionally on the background information $\mathcal{D}$:

$$\Pr(E \cup F \mid \mathcal{D}) = \Pr(E \mid \mathcal{D}) + \Pr(F \mid \mathcal{D}) - \Pr(E \cap F \mid \mathcal{D}), \qquad (2.1)$$

where the symbols "$\cup$" and "$\cap$" indicate respectively logical *disjunction* ("or") and *conjunction* ("and") of the two events.

Multiplicativity: For each pair of events E, F and conditionally on the background information $\mathcal{D}$:

$$\Pr(E \cap F \mid \mathcal{D}) = \Pr(F \mid E \cap \mathcal{D}) \times \Pr(E \mid \mathcal{D}). \qquad (2.2)$$

It is easy to show by simple counting[2] that these three rules hold for the urn model and then *a fortiori* for a generic event. The whole construction of

---

[1]Notice that alternative presentations of subjective probabilities directly in terms of betting odds have been proposed, e.g. notably by de Finetti (1974). However, this has the disadvantage of implicitly mixing the *quality* (i.e. the monetary sum the bettor can win or lose) and the *uncertainty* of the event being assessed. Thus, we prefer to follow the argument of Lindley (2006) and discuss subjective probabilities in comparison with the simple framework of the urn.

[2]For instance, to prove additivity it is sufficient to show that $\Pr(E \cup F \mid \mathcal{D})$ can be derived considering an urn with n balls, either red or white, and, at the same time, either plain or row. It is easy to count the proportion of red or plain balls as the the proportion of red balls plus the proportion of plain balls minus the proportion of red *and* plain balls (to avoid double counting), as in (2.1).

probability calculus is then derived by extending these properties, thus making the comparison to the urn standard just a theoretical device. For example, if we define E^c as the complement of E, the relationship

$$\Pr(E \mid \mathcal{D}) = 1 - \Pr(E^c \mid \mathcal{D}) \tag{2.3}$$

is easy to derive by combining (2.2) with convexity.

Interestingly, the rules described above are consistent with Kolmogorov's approach, which is generally regarded as the reference in probability calculus and is effectively the basis for the frequentist approach to statistical inference. Thus, it is perfectly possible to use subjective probabilities and apply the standard rules of probability calculus (Gillies, 2000).

One subtle difference, however, is that under the Bayesian approach, these rules can be *derived* (rather than *postulated* as axioms) from the fundamental assumption that defines "reasonable" behaviour of an individual facing uncertainty (Spiegelhalter et al., 2004). Crucially, reasonable (i.e. rational) behaviour of an individual is linked to this construction through the concept of *coherence*.

2.2.3   Coherence

The nature of the subjectivist paradigm is such that by definition the quantification of the degree of belief in a random event E is free, since each individual can derive a probability by comparing their degree of belief to the standard model. This probability is based on the relationship that they perceive with the event and that is not linked with repeatability under constant conditions of the experiment under analysis.

However, not only does this assessment of uncertainty need to conform with the rules of probability; it also has to be constructed in such a way that the individual's decisions based on it must not produce inconsistencies or irrational behaviour, e.g. taking a series of bets that the individual expressing the probabilistic judgement is certain to lose (de Finetti, 1974).

Example: incoherent definition of subjective probabilities

Define the odds *for* an event E as:

$$o(E) := \frac{\Pr(E)}{\Pr(E^c)} = \frac{\Pr(E)}{1 - \Pr(E)} \tag{2.4}$$

(implicitly discounting the common background information $\mathcal{D}$, in order to simplify the notation). Similarly, it is possible to define the odds *against* E as:

$$q(E) := \frac{1}{o(E)} = \frac{\Pr(E^c)}{\Pr(E)} = \frac{\Pr(E^c)}{1 - \Pr(E^c)},$$

and then verify the chain of equations:

$$o(E) = \frac{1}{q(E)} = q(E^c) = \frac{1}{o(E^c)}.$$

Consider now a bookmaker offering the following bets (Lindley, 2006).

Bet 1 The random event E is offered at odds against of $q_1 = 1 : 1$; in other words, if E obtains, then the bookmaker pays the wager s_1 multiplied by the odds against it (1, in this case). If, on the contrary E does not obtain (and therefore E^c does), the bookmaker wins the sum s_1.

Bet 2 The random event E^c is offered at odds against of $q_2 = 2 : 1$; in other words, if E^c obtains, then the bookmaker pays the wager s_2 multiplied by the odds against it (2, in this case). If, on the contrary E^c does not obtain, the bookmaker wins the the the sum s_2.

TABLE 2.1
The bookmaker's possible gain

Realised event	Bet 1	Bet 2	Total
E	$-q_1 s_1$	$+s_2$	$s_2 - q_1 s_1$
E^c	$+s_1$	$-q_2 s_2$	$s_1 - q_2 s_2$

The bookmaker's possible gains are described in Table 2.1, as functions of the event that actually obtains. If the punter places Bet 1 by paying a sum $s_1 = 3$ and Bet 2 by paying a sum $s_2 = 2$, it is easy to show that when E obtains, the bookmaker totals $(s_2 - q_1 s_1) = (2 - 3) = -1$, i.e. a loss of 1 monetary unit. Similarly, if E^c occurs, the bookmaker's gain is $(s_1 - q_2 s_2) = (3 - 4) = -1$, again a 1 monetary unit loss.

Such a bet is known as a *Dutch book*[3] and can be used to show how an incoherent definition of probabilities implies a behaviour that potentially leads to a certain loss. In fact, combining (2.4) with the other properties of odds, it is possible to show that the definition of the odds given by the bookmaker implies:

$$\Pr(E) = \frac{1}{1 + o(E)} = \frac{q(E)}{1 + q(E)} = \frac{1}{1 + 1} = \frac{1}{2}$$

and, at the same time that:

$$\Pr(E^c) = \frac{1}{1 + q(E^c)} = \frac{1}{1 + 2} = \frac{1}{3}.$$

---

[3]This terminology comes from the 1920–1930s and in particular from the work developed independently by Frank Ramsey and Bruno de Finetti. However, its etymology is still not clear.

Thus, the definition of subjective probabilities given by the bookmaker violates (2.3), since

$$\Pr(E) + \Pr(E^c) = \frac{1}{2} + \frac{1}{3} = \frac{5}{6} \neq 1,$$

which is against the fundamental rules of probability and therefore implies incoherence. The bookmaker then needs to re-assess the judgement of the uncertainty on E.

Incidentally, bookmakers typically define the odds so that the sum of the probabilities for the relevant events is greater than 1, as a fail-safe against the wagers.   □

In summary, under the subjectivist view, an individual is entitled to their own value of $\Pr(E)$. But once this probability has been assigned, in order to obtain a rational scheme of behaviour, the three fundamental rules of probability calculus and the other rules deriving from them constrain the individual to describe the uncertainty about events that are related to E using probabilities that are consistent with $\Pr(E)$.

In other words, individuals expressing subjective probabilities need to be coherent. Failure to do so, can lead to decision-making that is guaranteed to produce a certain loss (e.g., but not necessarily, in monetary terms). Thus, coherence and subjective probabilities generate a rational scheme for the measurement of uncertainty.

2.2.4   Bayes theorem

The Bayesian procedure can be viewed as a very effective way of formally representating the process of updating the degree of uncertainty about an event, as a consequence of the acquisition of additional information. This updating process is operationally given by the application of Bayes theorem.

Formally, the theorem is derived by the iterative application of multiplicativity. Consider two events A and B and the background information $\mathcal{D}$ (which again we assume constant and therefore do not explicitly include in the notation, for the sake of simplicity). By (2.2), the probability that A occurs, given that B has occurred is:

$$\Pr(A \mid B) \;\; = \;\; \frac{\Pr(B \cap A)}{\Pr(B)}. \qquad (2.5)$$

Suppose that the interest is in the probability that B occurs, conditionally on the fact that A has occurred. Using (2.2) again:

$$\Pr(B \mid A) \;\; = \;\; \frac{\Pr(A \cap B)}{\Pr(A)}. \qquad (2.6)$$

Finally, Bayes theorem is obtained by substituting (2.5) in (2.6):

$$\Pr(B \mid A) \;\; = \;\; \frac{\Pr(A \mid B) \times \Pr(B)}{\Pr(A)}. \qquad (2.7)$$

As mentioned earlier, the qualitative interpretation of Bayes theorem is particularly interesting. Every prior information on the occurrence of B is taken into account by means of the distribution $\Pr(B)$ and is then combined with the additional information (i.e. the fact that A obtains) that has become available, to update the current knowledge into the posterior distribution $\Pr(B \mid A)$.

An additional interesting feature of the Bayesian approach is that it allows a straightforward *sequential updating* of the uncertainty. In fact, if further additional evidence became available, e.g. in the form of the occurrence of a third event C, it would be possible to easily incorporate this extra information on the evaluation of the uncertainty about B by iteratively applying Bayes theorem:

$$\Pr(B \mid A \cap C) = \frac{\Pr(C \mid A \cap B) \times \Pr(B \mid A)}{\Pr(C \mid A)}.$$

In this case the posterior distribution given A is considered to be the current state of knowledge. In other words, the posterior distribution obtained after conditioning on A is used as the "new" prior distribution before the additional evidence C is observed. Uncertainty over B is then updated by including all the available information. To put it as Lindley (1972): "today's posterior is tomorrow's prior."

Example: Inverse probability

A typical application of Bayes theorem is the so called "inverse probability" analysis. Suppose for instance that the interest is in a diagnostic test T, whose possible outcomes with reference to a given disease are *positive* (which we indicate as "+") and *negative* ("−"). Let D (D^c) indicate the presence (absence) of the disease and suppose that the *sensitivity*

$$sens(T) := \Pr(+ \mid D) = 0.99$$

and the *specificity*:

$$spec(T) := \Pr(- \mid D^c) = 0.95,$$

of the test are known. Finally, suppose that the disease prevalence in the population is known to be 10%, i.e. $\Pr(D) = 0.1$.

What is the uncertainty about the possibility that an individual taking the test actually has the disease, if the test is positive? Intuitively, before we access the test result, and without any extra information, it is reasonable to assume that the probability that this patient has the disease is that of an individual selected at random from the population.

Often, the information about sensitivity of the test is misinterpreted to conclude that if the patient tests positive, then their probability of having the disease increases from the original value (0.1) to the sensitivity, 0.99 in this case. This error is often referred to as *prosecutor's fallacy*, a terminology derived from the legal jargon. Prosecutor's fallacy occurs when the probability of the evidence produced in court, conditionally on the hypothesis that the defendant is guilty, $\Pr(E \mid G)$, is misinterpreted by the prosecutor as the probability that the defendant is guilty given the evidence, $\Pr(G \mid E)$, which represents the actual objective of the legal evaluation, but that is in general numerically different.

In the case of the diagnostic test, instead of $\Pr(+ \mid D)$, the relevant probability is $\Pr(D \mid +)$, which can be easily computed from the available data, by using Baye's theorem:

$$
\begin{aligned}
\Pr(D \mid +) &= \frac{\Pr(+ \mid D) \times \Pr(D)}{\Pr(+ \mid D) \times \Pr(D) + \Pr(+ \mid D^c) \times \Pr(D^c)} \\
&= \frac{sens(T) \times \Pr(D)}{sens(T) \times \Pr(D) + [1 - spec(T)] \times [1 - \Pr(D)]} \\
&= \frac{0.99 \times 0.1}{0.99 \times 0.1 + 0.05 \times 0.9} = \frac{0.09}{1.135} = 0.667.
\end{aligned}
$$

As is obvious, the observation of the evidence (i.e. that the patient tests positive) does modify the initial uncertainty, by increasing the probability that the patient has the disease. However, sensitivity and specificity are weighted by the prevalence of the disease (which in this case is relatively low) and therefore the required probability is only 2/3. □

2.3 Bayesian (parametric) modelling

The implications of (2.7) can be extended to more complex statistical models, where instead of single events, we deal with random variables. In particular, we focus on so called "parametric" models, i.e. where the uncertainty about the observed random variable Y is represented by means of a probability distribution, indexed by a finite (set of) parameter(s) θ, which may be the object of the inference we want to draw. We indicate this probability distribution[4] with $p(y \mid \theta)$, to stress the dependence of the variable Y and its possible values y on the parameters θ.

Notice that, in general, rather than possessing some physical property, θ merely represents a convenient mathematical construction useful to simplify the formalisation of the statistical model (cfr. §2.3.1). Nevertheless, since it is not possible to observe them, within the Bayesian framework the parameters are considered to be random variables. Thus, they are associated with

---

[4]We use the symbol $\Pr(\cdot)$ to indicate the *probability* of a single event, as in §2.2, whereas we use the symbol $p(y)$ to describe the probability *distribution* associated with a random variable Y. Moreover, we consider the background information $\mathcal{D}$ as constant and therefore do not explicitly include it in the notation.

a suitable probability function, in order to describe the uncertainty, or in other terms the state of the available knowledge on them. This distribution is indicated by $p(\theta)$.

For the observed variables (the data), imperfect knowledge depends essentially on the sampling selection. Typically we assume that the data $\mathbf{y} = \{y_1, \ldots, y_n\}$ are a random sample of observations from a reference population, made up by $N > n$ units. The uncertainty on the observed variable is given by the fact that we only observe a single sample (*sampling variability*).

Conversely, the uncertainty about parameters is generated by our ignorance, or at most limited knowledge. Usually, we are not able to observe parameters, which typically represent latent, or hidden features of the data (more on this in §2.3.1). Consequently, we are not able to describe θ with certainty; we only have limited information about it, or maybe solely our subjective belief. We can use whatever information we have available about θ to define the *prior* distribution, $p(\theta)$.

One possible way to describe this prior knowledge consists in defining a parametric model, i.e. a probability distribution which is indexed by (a set of) "hyper-parameter(s)" ψ and that suitably represents the (subjective) current uncertainty (cfr. §5.3). In this case, it would be more appropriate to write the prior distribution as a function $p(\theta \mid \psi) = f(\psi)$, to stress this relationship. However, for the sake of simplicity, unless strictly necessary, we will use the notation $p(\theta)$ instead of $p(\theta \mid \psi)$, considering only implicitly the background information provided by ψ.

Bayesian inference is performed by applying (2.7) to compute:

$$p(\theta \mid y) = \frac{p(y \mid \theta) \times p(\theta)}{p(y)}. \tag{2.8}$$

The quantity $p(y \mid \theta)$ represents the *model for the observed data*. In particular, when viewed as a function of θ for the realised value of y, this is known as the *likelihood*, which we indicate as $\mathcal{L}(\theta)$.

The quantity $p(y)$ represents the *marginal* distribution of the observable variable Y and can be considered as a normalisation constant.

Finally, $p(\theta \mid y)$ is the *posterior* distribution, which is defined conditionally on the observed random variable $Y = y$. The denominator of (2.8) being a constant (with respect to θ), Bayes theorem is often reported as:

$$p(\theta \mid y) \propto p(y \mid \theta) \times p(\theta).$$

In the Bayesian approach, only one type of uncertainty exists: whether the quantity to be evaluated is represented by observable data or by an unobservable parameter; uncertainty is expressed by a probability distribution which suitably describes the level of (possibly, but not necessarily, subjective) knowledge about that quantity.

The relationships between the observable variable y and the parameter θ (and possibly the hyper-parameter ψ) might be better appreciated using the graphical representation of Directed Acyclic Graphs (DAGs; see Whittaker, 1990 and Gilks et al., 1996, or, for a less technical introduction, Edwards, 2000). In a DAG, the nodes (represented as circles) denote random quantities, while the arrows between the nodes represent stochastic dependencies.

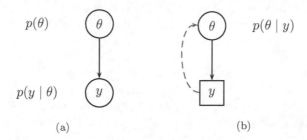

FIGURE 2.1
The DAG representation of (a) the data generating process; and (b) the probability updating process.

Figure 2.1(a) shows the alleged *data generating process*: the arrow leaving the node θ towards the node y means that the distribution of the observable variable depends (i.e. is conditional) on that of the parameter θ. Conversely, the *inferential process* is depicted in Figure 2.1(b). The variable Y is actually observed (i.e. it becomes *evidence* and is thus represented by means of a square, instead of by a circle); the evidence provided by this observation travels "against the arrows" of the DAG (the dashed line). This process of probability update is performed by means of the application of Bayes theorem.

2.3.1 Exchangeability and predictive inference

One of the most common assumptions underlying statistical models is that the observed data $\mathbf{y} = \{y_1, \ldots, y_n\}$ form an *independent and identically distributed* (*iid*) random sample. This is equivalent to assuming that, if the parameter θ actually had some physical meaning and its "true" value were known, then the observations would be conditionally independent:

$$p(y_1, \ldots, y_n \mid \theta) = \prod_{i=1}^{n} p(y_i \mid \theta). \tag{2.9}$$

If (2.9) is a reasonable assumption, it is possible to simplify the quantification of uncertainty about the observed data $(y_1, \ldots, y_n)$, since it is sufficient to analyse a single univariate distribution (considered to be the same conditionally on the unknown value of θ), instead of a n-variate joint distribution.

A more general concept, which proves less restrictive in many applied situations, is that the probabilistic structures of the single units are *similar* (rather than *identical*), with reference to some common generating process. This concept is generally known as *exchangeability* and it has strong connections with the Bayesian approach, thanks to the pioneering work of Bruno de Finetti (1974)[5].

Formally, a sequence of random variables $(y_1, \ldots, y_n)$ is judged as exchangeable if the degree of belief in the occurrence of that sequence, $be(y_1, \ldots, y_n)$, does not depend on the order with which the variables are observed. For example, if $n = 3$ binary variables are considered, the assumption of exchangeability implies that the probability of observing the outcome "1" twice and the outcome "0" once does not depend on the order. In other words, the person expressing the probabilistic assessment deems $\Pr(Y_1 = 1, Y_2 = 0, Y_3 = 1) = \Pr(Y_1 = 0, Y_2 = 1, Y_3 = 1) = \Pr(Y_1 = 1, Y_2 = 1, Y_3 = 0)$.

The general result proved by de Finetti is that the hypothesis of exchangeability implies that:

$$p(y_1, \ldots, y_n) = \int \prod_{i=1}^{n} p(y_i \mid \theta) p(\theta) \mathrm{d}\theta, \tag{2.10}$$

where θ is a continuous random parameter. Notice that (2.10) represents a generalisation of (2.9).

Figure 2.2 shows the difference between two samples of *iid* and exchangeable observations, in terms of a DAG. In the former case, the parameter generates the probability distribution of the observations and it is considered as a fixed quantity. Therefore, it is represented as a square in the DAG of Figure 2.2(a). On the contrary, in the case of exchangeable observations, the parameter is assumed to be a random variable (and it is therefore represented as a circle), associated with its own probability distribution. In both cases, the observations are conditionally independent, given (i.e. if we were able to observe the realised value of) θ. Nevertheless, the nature of the parameter is substantially different in the two cases.

The interpretation of (2.10) is that the degree of belief in the occurrence of the sequence of random variables $(y_1, \ldots, y_n)$, judged by the individual expressing it as exchangeable, can be derived by considering the observations as an *iid* sample that is drawn from a common distribution. This is indexed by a parameter, which in turn is considered to be a random variable associated with a probability distribution $p(\theta)$.

For de Finetti, the objective of inference is the assessment of the uncertainty on the observable variables, represented by $p(y_1, \ldots, y_n)$. As suggested earlier, in general θ has no real physical meaning and can be viewed as a convenient and abstract construction that is just useful to simplify the calculations. Thus, when analysed from left to right, (2.10) provides a justification of the

---

[5]de Finetti's theory on exchangeability as a means of justification for subjectivism dates back to the 1930s. However, his papers were almost exclusively published in his native Italian, which limited the diffusion of his ideas. Savage (1954) was probably the first to acknowledge de Finetti's work in the Anglo-Saxon literature.

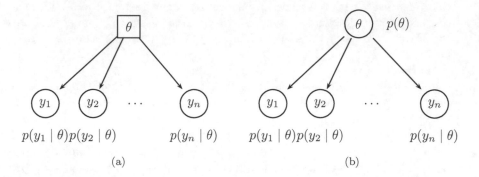

FIGURE 2.2
The DAG representation of: (a) a sample of *iid* observations; and (b) a sample of exchangeable observations. In both cases the observable variables depend on a parameter θ, which in case (a) is a fixed quantity, while in case (b) is a random variable associated with the distribution $p(\theta)$.

Bayesian procedure, in the sense that in order to quantify the uncertainty about the observable data it is convenient to think as a Bayesian by assuming exchangeability and the existence of a random parameter characterising the probability distribution of $\mathbf{y}$.

Obviously, the judgement of exchangeability does not necessarily hold in every situation; however, it can be partially relaxed by assuming a "conditional" version, where observations can be assumed to be similar, given the observed value of an extra variable (e.g. a covariate).

Moreover, from (2.10) it is possible to derive a *predictive* result on the observable variable. Suppose that y^* represents a future occurrence (or a value not yet observed in the current experiment) of the random phenomenon described by the information gathered by means of the sample $\mathbf{y}$. If we assume exchangeability for the augmented dataset $\mathbf{y}^* = \{\mathbf{y}, y^*\}$, we then have that:

$$p(y^* \mid \mathbf{y}) = \frac{p(y^*, \mathbf{y})}{p(\mathbf{y})} \qquad \text{(by definition of conditional probability)}$$

$$= \frac{\int p(y^* \mid \theta) p(\mathbf{y} \mid \theta) p(\theta) \mathrm{d}\theta}{p(\mathbf{y})} \qquad \text{(by exchangeability)}$$

$$= \frac{\int p(y^* \mid \theta) p(\theta \mid \mathbf{y}) p(\mathbf{y}) \mathrm{d}\theta}{p(\mathbf{y})} \qquad \text{(applying Bayes theorem)}$$

$$= \int p(y^* \mid \theta) p(\theta \mid \mathbf{y}) \mathrm{d}\theta. \qquad (2.11)$$

Equation (2.11) is meaningful only under the assumption that the new realisation y^* is exchangeable with the ones that have already been observed, $\mathbf{y}$. The quantity $p(y^* \mid \mathbf{y})$ is known as the *(posterior) predictive distribution*.

Figure 2.3 shows the concept of predictive distribution in terms of a DAG. The variables y and y^* are generated by the same random process, which is governed by the parameter θ, associated with a suitable prior distribution, $p(\theta)$. Once $Y = y$ is observed, the uncertainty about the parameter is updated into the posterior distribution $p(\theta \mid y)$, which in turn is used to infer about the future realisation of the variable y^*.

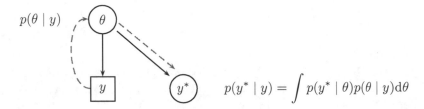

$$p(y^* \mid y) = \int p(y^* \mid \theta) p(\theta \mid y) \mathrm{d}\theta$$

FIGURE 2.3
A DAG representation of the concept of predictive distribution.

2.3.2 Inference on the posterior distribution

Although we reiterate that, technically, the parameter θ can be seen as an abstract concept needed to produce a simple evaluation of the uncertainty on the observable variables, it is often possible to devise a statistical model in which the parameters assume some real meaning. For example, this is the case when the parameters represent some unobservable "population" characteristics that may become relevant in themselves. In those cases, inference on the posterior distribution becomes, at least partly, the actual objective of the analysis.

The frequentist approach considers the parameter as a physical property of the data, possessing an unknown but fixed value and uses the observed data as random quantities (randomness being induced by sampling variability) for the inferential process. In order to estimate the "true" value of the parameter, frequentist procedures use an estimator (the most important being the *Maximum Likelihood Estimator*, MLE), which is a function of the data: $\hat{\theta} = t(\mathbf{y})$.

On the contrary, the Bayesian procedure considers the data as fixed quantities. This happens because once the data are observed, they become evidence and at that point there is no uncertainty on their realised value. The inferential process is performed by means of a function of the parameter, conditionally on the observed data, i.e. the posterior distribution $p(\theta \mid \mathbf{y})$.

Goodman (1999) argues that Bayesian inference has an *inductive* nature: starting from the observed evidence, the probabilistic judgement on the parameters is updated. This procedure is in contrast with the *deductive* frequentist approach, which evaluates the plausibility of the observed data, conditionally on some fixed value for the parameters (cfr. Figure 2.4).

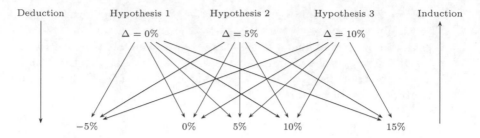

FIGURE 2.4

Deduction fixes the value of the reference hypotheses and evaluates probabilistically the plausibility of the observed data; on the other hand, inductive inference is based on the observed information (data and background knowledge) to infer about unobserved hypotheses. Adapted from Goodman (1999).

Example: Inference on the probability of survival after a risky operation

Consider a situation where a patient undergoes a risky surgical operation. We assume a very simple (and even more unrealistic!) model where the possible outcomes of the operation are a success, known to happen with probability $p = 0.2$, or a failure (which of course has a probability of $1-p = 0.8$). Following the operation, the patient can either survive a long enough amount of time, beyond which they are deemed to be cured, or die. We indicate the probability of survival with θ and we assume that if the operation was successful, then $\theta = 0.9$; however, if the operation failed, then the patient has a lower chance of surviving: $\theta = 0.3$. The actual observation is a variable x_i taking values 1 if the i-th patient survives and 0 otherwise. Figure 2.5 shows a graphical representation of the problem.

Under this specification, the unknown parameter θ is a discrete variable with only two possible values and its prior distribution can be described by the following conditions: $\Pr(\theta = 0.3) = 0.8$ and $\Pr(\theta = 0.9) = 0.2$. Suppose that a total of $n = 10$ patients are observed, of whom $y = \sum_{i=1}^{10} x_i = 7$ are known to survive the operation. What is the updated probability distribution of the chance of survival θ?

In this case, a reasonable model for the observed data is $y \mid \theta \sim$ Binomial(θ, n), so that

$$p(y \mid \theta) = \binom{n}{y} \theta^y (1 - \theta)^{(n-y)}$$
$$\propto \theta^y (1 - \theta)^{(n-y)},$$

which as a function of θ represents the likelihood $\mathcal{L}(\theta)$. Considering the avail-

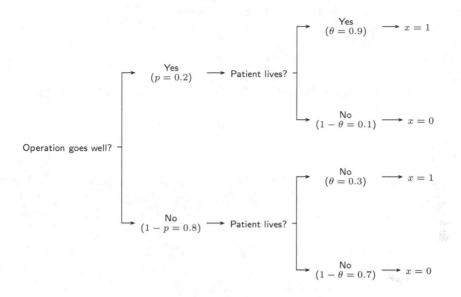

FIGURE 2.5
A graphical representation of the problem of survival after a risky operation.
Reading the graph from left to right shows the data-generating process: the
outcome of the operation determines the distribution of the probability of
survival, which in turn determines the observed patient outcome (survival or
death). Reading the graph from right to left shows the inferential process:
once the patient outcome is known, it is possible to identify the most likely
"cause", given the probabilistic structure assumed in the model.

able data, it is possible to compute:

$$\mathcal{L}(0.3) = 0.3^7 \times 0.7^3 = 0.00007, \quad \text{and}$$
$$\mathcal{L}(0.9) = 0.9^7 \times 0.1^3 = 0.00047.$$

Combining these with the prior distribution we can produce the posterior as:

$$\Pr(\theta = 0.3 \mid y = 7, n = 10) = \frac{0.00007 \times 0.8}{(0.00047 \times 0.2) + (0.00007 \times 0.8)} = 0.374,$$

and

$$\Pr(\theta = 0.9 \mid y = 7, n = 10) = \frac{0.00047 \times 0.2}{(0.00047 \times 0.2) + (0.00007 \times 0.8)} = 0.626.$$

The observation of a large proportion of surviving patients has the effect
of shifting our prior belief on θ being equal to 0.9 from a value of only 0.2

to a value of over 0.6 after the evidence becomes available. In other words, after seeing the data, it looks more likely that the operation tends to go well than we had originally thought. This is perhaps an indication that our prior knowledge was not well calibrated.   □

Although the posterior distribution provides in itself all the information on the parameter after having observed the data, it is generally useful to summarize it through some suitable synthetic indicators.

Point estimates

Similarly to what happens in classical statistics, typical point estimators are the mode, the median and the mean of the posterior distribution. These estimators are calculated according to the usual definitions provided in the statistical literature (e.g. in Mood et al. 1993).

For instance, the posterior mean is calculated as: $E(\theta \mid y) = \int \theta p(\theta \mid y) d\theta$. Similarly, we can calculate the posterior median as the value that separates the highest half of the posterior distribution from the lowest half: θ_{med} such that $p(\theta < \theta_{med} \mid y) = \frac{1}{2}$, or the posterior mode as the value(s) associated with the maximum frequency (or with the maximum density in case of a continuous variable): $\theta^* = \arg\max_\Theta p(\theta \mid y)$ – this kind of estimator is often referred to as *Maximum A Posteriori* (MAP). In addition to location summaries, it is possible to consider variability indicators, as for instance the posterior variance: $Var(\theta \mid y) = \int [\theta - E(\theta \mid y)]^2 p(\theta \mid y) d\theta$.

Credibility intervals

The parallel with the classical approach extends to interval estimation. However, the philosophy underlying the Bayesian approach is completely different. In the frequentist framework, a $100 \times (1-\alpha)\%$ confidence interval (CI) suggests that *if we were able to repeat the same experiment, under the same conditions for a large number M of times*, then the real value of θ will fall out of that interval only $100 \times \alpha\%$ of the times. This convoluted statement is *not* equivalent to asserting that the probability that θ lies in the CI is $100 \times (1-\alpha)\%$, since the parameter is considered as a fixed, unknown value, not as a random variable. Moreover, the definition of the frequentist CI does not help clarify what we can say about the *current* experiment (cfr. Table 2.2).

Conversely, assuming that θ has some context-specific meaning (as opposed to being just a mathematical device to simplify the estimation of the joint distribution of the observed variables $\mathbf{y}$), within the Bayesian framework a confidence interval CI explicitly indicates the probability $\Pr(\theta \in CI \mid y)$. This is made possible by the fact that the parameter of interest is associated with a probability distribution, which allows one to make probabilistic statements and to take the underlying uncertainty into account. No reference is made to

TABLE 2.2

The basic differences between the frequentist and the Bayesian approach.
Adapted from: Luce and O'Hagan (2003)

Frequentist	Bayesian
Nature of probability	
The limiting long-run frequency on a large number of identical replications of the experiment at hand	The personal degree of belief on the realization of the specific outcome under study in the experiment at hand
Nature of parameters	
Unknown, unrepeatable quantities	Non observable quantities, subjected to their own variability, given the knowledge of the experimenter
Nature of inference	
Does not (although it appears to) make probabilistic statements about the parameters of interest	Makes direct probability statements about parameters with respect to the current experiment
Example	
We reject this hypothesis at the 5% level of significance:	*The probability that this hypothesis is true is 0.05:*
If the experimental condition were held constant and we could observe an infinite number of equivalent samples, in 5% of the cases the hypothesis would be rejected (but what happens to the observed sample?)	In the actually available sample, the data suggest a weak evidence to the hypothesis: $\Pr(H_0 \mid \text{data}) = 0.05$

long run replications of the experiment. To highlight this difference, Bayesian intervals are generally referred to as "*credibility*" intervals.

Without the need of approximations or convoluted statements, it is in theory straightforward to compute a credibility interval by solving the equation:

$$\Pr(\theta \in \text{CI} \mid y) = \int_{\text{CI}} p(\theta \mid y)\mathrm{d}\theta = 1 - \alpha \tag{2.12}$$

for any level α of interest.

Technically, a credibility interval is not necessarily unique, since there might be many possible solutions to equation (2.12). In principle, the optimal solution is to consider the interval with minimum length, typically termed a *Highest Posterior Density* (HPD) interval (Bernardo and Smith, 1999). The actual computation of this interval can be cumbersome, especially when the posterior distribution is highly skewed or, even worse, characterised by multi-modality. However, in many applied cases it is possible to solve the problem operationally by computing the 2.5th and the 97.5th percentiles of the posterior distribution. The interval whose extremes are given by these two values contains 95% of the probability mass. For (approximately) symmetrical distributions, this is effectively identical with the HPD interval.

2.4 Choosing prior distributions and Bayesian computation

Arguably, the most controversial aspect of a Bayesian analysis is represented by the choice of the prior distribution, a suitable mathematical model which could well describe the nature of the parameters and the experimenter's uncertainty about their values. As suggested above, the definition of the prior distribution should be informed by whatever knowledge is available on the parameters and ideally the experimenter should be able to describe this information by means of some mathematical form.

This, however, can be quite a difficult task and, in general, there can be no standard probability distribution that exactly quantifies the qualitative information available to the individual performing the analysis. Moreover, the choice of the prior distribution has been until recently associated with almost insurmountable practical problems, given the generally great computational difficulties encountered with all but trivial models.

In the next sections, we review the main types of prior distributions and discuss the computational issues arising from their application.

2.4.1 Vague priors

Sometimes the experimenter has only a minimal knowledge of the features of the data generating process that are represented by the parameters of the model. In these circumstances, it might be reasonable to use a vague (often, but quite controversially, referred to as "non informative") prior, which basically does not favour any of the possible values that the parameter θ can take on. Alternative terminologies to describe this kind of prior distribution are "flat," "dispersed" or "minimally informative."

In fact, the original works of Bayes and Laplace were based on flat priors, on the grounds of the "principle of insufficient reason". Laplace argued that unless a strong belief can be placed on some particular values of the parameters in a model, it makes sense to use a prior that encodes complete ignorance and assumes that each of the values be equally likely before observing the evidence. This choice, which typically amounts to assuming a Uniform prior distribution, lets "the data speak for themselves" and therefore, at least in theory, limits the subjectivism associated with the application of Bayes theorem.

If the vague prior distribution is chosen to be Uniform, which implies $p(\theta) = k$ for a given constant k, then the posterior distribution is simply obtained as

$$p(\theta \mid y) = \frac{p(y \mid \theta)p(\theta)}{p(y)}$$

$$= \frac{k \times p(y \mid \theta)}{\int k \times p(y \mid \theta)\mathrm{d}\theta}$$

$$= \frac{p(y \mid \theta)}{\int p(y \mid \theta)\mathrm{d}\theta} = \frac{\mathcal{L}(\theta)}{\int \mathcal{L}(\theta)\mathrm{d}\theta}.$$

Thus, under a Uniform prior, the posterior distribution is computed by normalising the likelihood function, which makes clear why Bayesian analyses based on flat priors are essentially identical with maximum likelihood estimations (in particular, the posterior mode is identical with the MLE).

Example: Estimating the proportion of female births in Paris

We consider here the famous data analysed by Laplace on the number of female births in Paris. In 1710, John Arbuthnot, a Scottish medical doctor with a passion for mathematics, analysed data on christening recorded in London between 1629 and 1710 to conclude that males were born at a "significantly" greater rate than females. This being somehow against the assumption of equal probability for the two sexes, he deduced that divine providence accounted for it, because males die young more often than females.

Laplace analysed similar data collected in Paris from 1745 to 1770. He observed a total of $y = 241\,945$ girls born out of a total of $n = 493\,527$ babies and was interested in estimating the probability of a female birth, θ. Laplace based his analysis on a reasonable Binomial model for the data: $y \mid \theta \sim \text{Binomial}(\theta, n)$ and pragmatically assigned a Uniform distribution in $[0; 1]$ to θ: $p(\theta) = 1$.

With these assumptions, the posterior distribution is:

$$p(\theta \mid y) = \frac{\binom{n}{y}\theta^y(1-\theta)^{(n-y)}}{\int_0^1 \binom{n}{y}\theta^y(1-\theta)^{(n-y)}\mathrm{d}\theta}.$$

In his paper, Bayes had already managed to evaluate the integral in the denominator as $1/(n+1)$, and therefore

$$p(\theta \mid y) = (n+1)\binom{n}{y}\theta^y(1-\theta)^{(n-y)}$$

$$= \frac{(n+1)n!}{(n-y)!y!}\theta^y(1-\theta)^{(n-y)}$$

$$= \frac{(n+1)!}{(n-y)!y!}\theta^y(1-\theta)^{(n-y)}. \tag{2.13}$$

Since the gamma function is defined as $\Gamma(k) = (k-1)!$ it is possible to rewrite (2.13) as

$$p(\theta \mid y) = \frac{\Gamma(n+2)}{\Gamma(n-y+1)\Gamma(y+1)}\theta^y(1-\theta)^{(n-y)},$$

which happens to be the density of a Beta random variable with parameters $\alpha = (y+1)$ and $\beta = (n-y+1)$. So, in other words, $\theta \mid y \sim \text{Beta}(\alpha, \beta)$.

Using the mathematical properties of this density, it can be shown that:

$$\text{E}(\theta \mid y) = \frac{\alpha}{\alpha+\beta} \qquad \text{and} \qquad \text{Var}(\theta \mid y) = \frac{\alpha\beta}{(\alpha+\beta)^2(\alpha+\beta+1)}, \qquad (2.14)$$

i.e. a Beta random variable has mean and variance defined in terms of the parameters (α, β) according to (2.14). Consequently, the analysis can be completed by computing the summary statistics, for instance

$$\text{E}(\theta \mid y) = \frac{y+1}{n+2} = \frac{241\,946}{493\,529} = 0.49024,$$

which is effectively identical with the MLE $\hat{\theta} = 0.49025$. Laplace also calculated that the posterior probability that $\theta \geq 0.5 = 1.15 \times 10^{-42}$ and concluded that he was "morally certain" that it was in fact less than 0.5, in accordance with Arbuthnot's finding.   □

Despite their apparent usefulness in providing a simple form for the prior, there are several problems with choosing vague formulations. First, they do not necessarily encode the prior information available to the experimenter. There are indeed cases where prior knowledge is poor, but in many applied cases, either hard evidence (perhaps provided by previously run studies) or expert opinions (given by extensive theoretical insight into the subject matter) are available and should be used to perform the Bayesian analysis.

Second, it is possible that vague priors be *improper* (i.e. they do not integrate to 1 and therefore do not define a probability distribution, in violation of the fundamental rules of probability). This happens, for example, when the support of the parameter is the entire real line. For instance, if we assume a Uniform prior for the parameter θ, representing the mean of a Normal distribution, then $\int_{-\infty}^{+\infty} p(\theta)\mathrm{d}\theta = \infty$. This has two major problems: the first one is that it is not possible to give a clear interpretation of the qualitative meaning of the prior, since it does not represent a probability distribution. Moreover, it is possible that starting with an improper prior even in light of the observed evidence the posterior distribution is improper too. In that case, the inference produced by the Bayesian analysis is clearly unreliable.

Third, even when proper, vague priors are not invariant to transformation. This is not ideal since assuming ignorance on θ has exactly the same qualitative meaning as assuming ignorance on any transformation $\phi = g(\theta)$. However, the mathematical construction linked with vague priors is such that, generally, Uniform priors on one scale are not Uniform on another. By simply applying the rules for the change of variable, it is easy to see that vague information on the θ scale is not the same as having vague information on the $\phi = \exp(\theta)$ scale. The prior for ϕ, derived as

$$p(\phi) = \left| \frac{d}{d\phi} \log(\phi) \right| = \frac{1}{\phi},$$

is not flat, as shown in Figure 2.6.

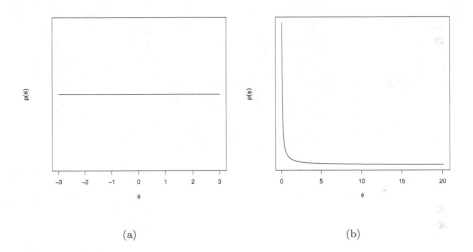

(a)   (b)

FIGURE 2.6
Lack of invariance to transformations for a flat prior: on the θ scale in panel (a) the prior distribution is Uniform. However, the corresponding prior for a transformation $\exp(\theta)$, shown in panel (b), is clearly not flat.

A special class of "non informative" priors that (at least for one-dimensional parameters) are invariant to transformations is represented by the so-called *Jeffreys priors* (Jeffreys, 1961). These are defined as

$$p(\theta) \propto \mathcal{I}(\theta)^{1/2},$$

where

$$\mathcal{I}(\theta) = -\mathrm{E}_{Y|\theta} \left[\frac{\partial^2 \log p(y \mid \theta)}{\partial \theta^2} \right] = \mathrm{E}_{Y|\theta} \left[\left(\frac{\partial \log p(y \mid \theta)}{\partial \theta} \right)^2 \right]$$

is the *Fisher information*, a measure of the amount of information that the observable random quantity y carries on the parameter θ.

Together with invariance, the main feature of Jeffreys priors is that, because of their mathematical properties, they force the influence of the prior to be the same as that of the data, for which reason they are characterised as "non informative."

To see this, consider for example a model $y \sim \text{Binomial}(\theta, n)$. Under this distributional assumption

$$\log p(y \mid \theta) = y \log(\theta) + (n - y) \log(1 - \theta)$$

and thus the first and second derivatives are

$$\frac{\partial \log p(y \mid \theta)}{\partial \theta} = \frac{y}{\theta} - \frac{n - y}{1 - \theta}$$

and

$$\frac{\partial^2 \log p(y \mid \theta)}{\partial \theta^2} = -\frac{y}{\theta^2} - \frac{n - y}{(1 - \theta)^2},$$

respectively. Because in the Binomial model $E_{Y\mid\theta}(Y) = n\theta$, it is easy to see that $\mathcal{I}(\theta) = n/(1 - \theta)$ and therefore Jeffreys prior is defined as

$$
\begin{aligned}
p(\theta) \quad &\propto \quad \mathcal{I}(\theta)^{1/2} \\
&= \quad -E_{Y\mid\theta} \left[-\frac{Y}{\theta^2} - \frac{n - Y}{(1 - \theta)^2} \right]^{1/2} \\
&= \quad \left[\frac{n\theta}{\theta^2} + \frac{n(1 - \theta)}{(1 - \theta)^2} \right]^{1/2} \\
&= \quad \left[\frac{n}{\theta(1 - \theta)} \right]^{1/2} \quad \propto \quad \theta^{-1/2}(1 - \theta)^{-1/2},
\end{aligned}
$$

which, as is possible to see by comparison with (2.13), is a Beta distribution with parameters $(0.5, 0.5)$.

Intuitively, the information provided by Binomial data is the least when θ is close to 0.5. In fact, for $\theta = 0.5$, $\text{Var}_{Y\mid\theta}(Y) = \theta(1-\theta)/n$ is at the maximum. Conversely, when θ is near the extremes (i.e. close to 0 or 1), the data variance is at the minimum level, and therefore the data provide the highest impact over the prior.

"Non informative" Jeffreys priors compensate for this by placing more mass near the extremes of the range, as shown in Figure 2.7. Thus, whatever the value of the parameter, the prior distribution and the likelihood have effectively the same weight in the resulting inference. For this reason, they are sometimes referred to as "objective" priors.

Apart from the lack of invariance, Jeffreys priors share the limitations of the vague specifications described above, particularly with respect to improper distributions. Moreover, it is generally difficult to derive a Jeffreys formulation for multivariate parameters.

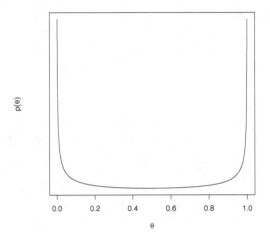

FIGURE 2.7
Jeffreys prior for θ, the parameter representing the probability of success in a binomial model, corresponding to a Beta$(0.5, 0.5)$ distribution.

2.4.2 Conjugate priors

A special type of prior that presents several computational advantages is that of *conjugate* models (Raiffa and Schlaifer, 1961).

A prior distribution $p(\theta \mid \psi) = f(\psi)$, as a function of the (set of) hyper-parameter(s) ψ is said to be conjugated for the data model $p(y \mid \theta)$ if the posterior distribution $p(\theta \mid y) = f(\psi^*)$ belongs to the same family of probability distributions f. In this case, the update from the prior to the posterior only involves the hyper-parameters, which are modified from ψ to ψ^*.

Technically, a conjugate prior distribution can be identified by studying the likelihood function and recognising that it is equivalent (or at least proportional) to a particular probability distribution. For instance, in the Binomial model the likelihood is $\mathcal{L}(\theta) = \theta^y (1 - \theta)^{(n-y)}$, which, as suggested above, when interpreted as a function of θ for fixed y is the *kernel* (i.e. the part of the density function that depends only on its argument) of a Beta distribution with parameters $(y + 1, n - y + 1)$.

Thus, applying Bayes theorem using a Beta prior distribution with hyper-parameters (α, β) will give

$$
\begin{aligned}
p(\theta \mid y) \quad &\propto \quad \mathcal{L}(\theta) \times p(\theta) \\
&\propto \quad \text{Beta}(y+1, n-y+1) \times \text{Beta}(\alpha, \beta) \\
&\propto \quad \left[\theta^y (1-\theta)^{n-y}\right] \times \left[\theta^{\alpha-1}(1-\theta)^{\beta-1}\right] \\
&= \quad \theta^{y+\alpha-1}(1-\theta)^{n-y+\beta-1},
\end{aligned}
$$

which is the kernel of a $\text{Beta}(y+\alpha, n-y+\beta)$ distribution. Consequently, the posterior distribution is still in the same functional form and the update process from prior to posterior only involves a change in the hyper-parameters, which are modified from (α, β) to $(y+\alpha, n-y+\beta)$ to incorporate the effect of the observed data.

Table 2.3 shows some common conjugate models — cfr. Bernardo and Smith (1999) for a taxonomic account of conjugated families. Throughout the table, the parameter of interest is indicated by θ.

Example: Conjugate prior for a Normal model with known variance

Consider a sample $\mathbf{y} = (y_1, \ldots, y_n)$ made by $n = 30$ observations on the weight at birth (in grams) for each baby (the complete dataset is available at `http://data.princeton.edu/wws509/datasets/#births`). The interest is in the estimation of the population average weight at birth, θ. We assume that the observed weights can be modelled as $y_i \mid \theta, \sigma^2 \sim \text{Normal}(\theta, \sigma^2)$, i.e.

$$
p(y_i \mid \theta, \sigma^2) = \frac{1}{\sqrt{2\pi}\sigma} \exp\left(-\frac{1}{2\sigma^2}(y_i - \theta)^2\right).
$$

To simplify matters, we assume that the population variance σ^2 is a known constant, for instance $\sigma = 650$ grams. Notice that it is generally easier to form a guess on the standard deviation scale, than it is on the variance. However, given the deterministic relationship linking the two, for any value (distribution) on the σ scale, a value (distribution) on the σ^2 scale will be automatically induced.

A conjugate analysis of this model considers a prior distribution of the form $\theta \sim \text{Normal}(\mu_0, \sigma_0^2)$. In general, it is possible to encode "minimal information" in this prior by defining a distribution centred around 0 and with large variance, e.g. $\mu_0 = 0$, $\sigma_0^2 = 10000$. The choice of the value for σ_0 to induce a minimally informative prior depends on the scale of the parameter. A standard deviation of 1000 can be large enough in some cases, but it could be much more informative in other situations.

In the present case, however, such a prior would be quite unreasonable: in fact, the population average weight at birth *must* be a positive variable and it physically cannot exceed some maximum threshold. Thus, it is just absurd to model prior knowledge by assuming that, before observing any data, our uncertainty on this variable is suitably represented by a distribution which

TABLE 2.3

Some relevant conjugated models. Throughout the table, the parameter of interest is indicated by θ. Additional parameters might characterise a given model, but might not represent the main focus of the inferential analysis (e.g. sometimes it is assumed that the variance σ^2 of a Normal model is less interesting than the mean)

Data model	Prior distribution	Posterior distribution	Notes
$\mathbf{y}\mid\theta, \sigma^2 \sim \text{Normal}(\theta, \sigma^2)$	$\theta \sim \text{Normal}(\mu_0, \sigma_0^2)$	$\theta\mid\mathbf{y} \sim \text{Normal}(\mu_1, \sigma_1^2)$	$\mu_1 = \dfrac{\frac{\mu_0}{\sigma_0^2} + \frac{n\bar{y}}{\sigma^2}}{\frac{1}{\sigma_0^2} + \frac{n}{\sigma^2}}$ $\sigma_1^2 = \dfrac{1}{\frac{1}{\sigma_0^2} + \frac{n}{\sigma^2}}$ $\bar{y} = \frac{1}{n}\sum_{i=1}^{n} y_i$
$\mathbf{y}\mid\theta \sim \text{Poisson}(\theta)$	$\theta \sim \text{Gamma}(\alpha, \beta)$	$\theta\mid\mathbf{y} \sim \text{Gamma}(\alpha^*, \beta^*)$	$\alpha^* = \alpha + s$ $\beta^* = \beta + n$ $s = \sum_{i=1}^{n} y_i$
$\mathbf{y}\mid\nu, \theta \sim \text{Gamma}(\nu, \theta)$	$\theta \sim \text{Gamma}(\alpha, \beta)$	$\theta\mid\mathbf{y} \sim \text{Gamma}(\alpha^*, \beta^*)$	$\alpha^* = \alpha + \nu$ $\beta^* = \beta + s$ $s = \sum_{i-1}^{n} y_i$
$\mathbf{y}\mid\theta \sim \text{Binomial}(n, \theta)$	$\theta \sim \text{Beta}(\alpha, \beta)$	$\theta\mid\mathbf{y} \sim \text{Beta}(\alpha^*, \beta^*)$	$\alpha^* = \alpha + s$ $\beta^* = \beta + n - s$ $s = \sum_{i=1}^{n} y_i$
$\mathbf{y}\mid\theta \sim \text{Exponential}(\theta)$	$\theta \sim \text{Gamma}(\alpha, \beta)$	$\theta\mid\mathbf{y} \sim \text{Gamma}(\alpha^*, \beta^*)$	$\alpha^* = \alpha + n$ $\beta^* = \beta + n\bar{y}$ $\bar{y} = \frac{1}{n}\sum_{i=1}^{n} y_i$
$\mathbf{y}\mid\mu, \frac{1}{\theta} \sim \text{Normal}\left(\mu, \frac{1}{\theta}\right)$	$\theta \sim \text{Gamma}(\alpha, \beta)$	$\theta\mid\mathbf{y} \sim \text{Gamma}(\alpha^*, \beta^*)$	$\alpha^* = \alpha + \frac{n}{2}$ $\beta^* = \beta + \frac{S}{2}$ $S = \sum_{i=1}^{n}(y_i - \mu)^2$

has mean equal to 0 and effectively not favouring any of the possible values in all the real line, i.e. the interval $(-\infty; +\infty)$.

Consequently, while it is possible that we do not have a clear idea of the actual value for θ and the attached uncertainty, it is necessary to assume reasonable values for (μ_0, σ_0^2), even to identify lack of precise information. For example, we could set $\mu_0 = 3000$ grams and still use a reasonably large standard deviation, for example $\sigma = 3000$.

Notice that, technically, this model would still allow negative birth weights, although with low probability. In real applications, this is not an ideal feature and the model should be modified (e.g. by using truncation, or a different data and prior distribution). Nevertheless, the impact of this feature of the final inference is not very high in this particular case and therefore this model is acceptable (although not ideal).

As is possible to see from Table 2.3, the posterior distribution is simply computed by updating the parameters of the Normal prior. The observed value for the sample average is in this case $\bar{y} = 3123.367$ and therefore $\mu_1 = 3123.174$ grams and $\sigma_1 = 118.5805$ grams. The posterior mean is effectively identical with the MLE $\bar{y} = 3123.367$ grams, to confirm the minimal impact of the prior. Moreover, the posterior distribution has a much smaller standard deviation than the prior, which is due to the data observed.

In the case of the Normal conjugate model with known variance, it is also easy to compute the predictive distribution for a new observation y^*. In fact,

$$
\begin{aligned}
p(y^* \mid \mathbf{y}) &= \int p(y^* \mid \theta) p(\theta \mid \mathbf{y}) \mathrm{d}\theta \\
&= \int \mathrm{Normal}(\theta, \sigma^2) \times \mathrm{Normal}(\mu_1, \sigma_1^2) \mathrm{d}\theta \\
&\propto \int \exp\left(-\frac{1}{2\sigma^2}(y^* - \theta)^2\right) \times \exp\left(-\frac{1}{2\sigma_1^2}(\theta - \mu_1)^2\right) \mathrm{d}\theta.
\end{aligned}
$$

Simple algebra allows to show that this produces a Normal distribution with mean μ_1 and variance $(\sigma^2 + \sigma_1^2)$.

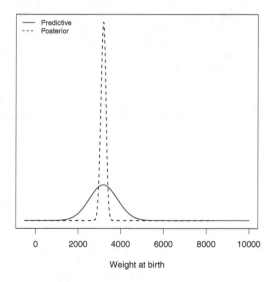

FIGURE 2.8
The posterior distribution $p(\theta \mid \mathbf{y})$ (dashed line) and the predictive distributions (solid line) for a new observations $p(y^* \mid \mathbf{y})$. The two distributions are both centred around the posterior mean μ_1, but the predictive distribution has a much larger variability.

Figure 2.8 shows both the posterior and the predictive distributions; as seems reasonable, the best guess for a new observation is based on the current level of knowledge (i.e. the average of the weight at birth, considering the information provided by the observed sample). However, since y^* is not observed, there is more uncertainty over its actual realisation and therefore the variance of the predictive is much larger than that of the posterior distribution. □

Example: Informative conjugate prior for Binomial data

Suppose that as part of a cancer screening programme, $n = 32$ screening kits are sent to eligible residents within a single postcode sector, of which only $y = 18$ are returned to the local health centre. A reasonable model for these data is again $y \mid \theta \sim \text{Binomial}(\theta, n)$, where θ represents the underlying population average response (screening uptake probability) in that given geographical area.

Suppose further that (for instance from historical data on the same postcode sector), the probability that a patient returns their kit has been estimated to be between 40 and 80%. The main idea of the Bayesian paradigm is to formally include this extra information in the analysis. This can be achieved by encoding it into the prior distribution.

One simple possibility is to create an "informative" conjugate prior; according to Table 2.3, this amounts to assuming that the functional form is $\theta \mid \alpha, \beta \sim \text{Beta}(\alpha, \beta)$, for suitable values of (α, β) that encode the available level of information. In other words, we need to find suitable values of (α, β) for which most of the probability mass for θ is concentrated in the interval $[0.4; 0.8]$. This can be obtained for example by assuming that $\text{E}(\theta) := \mu = 0.6$ and $\text{Var}(\theta) := \sigma^2 = 0.01$.

Using the mathematical properties of the Beta distribution and solving (2.14) for α and β gives:

$$\alpha = \mu \left[\frac{\mu(1-\mu)}{\sigma^2} - 1 \right] \quad \text{and} \quad \beta = (1-\mu) \left[\frac{\mu(1-\mu)}{\sigma^2} - 1 \right], \quad (2.15)$$

which in this case leads to $\alpha = 13.8$ and $\beta = 9.2$.

Figure 2.9 shows this prior distribution (the solid curve). As is possible to see, we are assigning a positive degree of belief to most of the support of θ (i.e. the interval $[0, 1]$). However, values around 0.6 are more likely than the others, while extreme values (e.g. less than 0.3 or greater than 0.9) are considered to be much less likely (or virtually impossible) and therefore are associated with low (or nearly zero) prior probability. As requested, most of the mass is contained in $[0.4; 0.8]$.

The observed evidence can be combined with this information to produce the posterior distribution $\theta \mid y \sim \text{Beta}(\alpha^*, \beta^*)$, with $\alpha^* = \alpha + y = 31.8$ and $\beta^* = \beta + n - y = 23.2$. Since this is a standard probability distribution, it is possible to compute analytically the relevant summary statistics of the posterior distribution; for instance, the posterior mean can be calculated at 0.5781 and a 95% credible interval is $[0.4466; 0.7043]$.

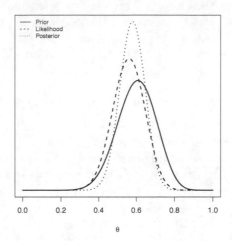

FIGURE 2.9
The graph shows the prior distribution (solid line) $\theta \mid \alpha, \beta \sim \text{Beta}(13.8, 9.2)$. This distribution encodes the assumption that most of the probability mass is in the interval $[0.4; 0.8]$. Also shown are the likelihood function and the posterior distribution. The latter can be seen as a compromise between the prior information and that provided by the observed evidence.

A standard frequentist analysis would proceed to compute the MLE and then a 95% confidence interval, typically by using an approximation to the Normal distribution, to produce an estimated uptake probability $\hat{\theta} = 0.5625$ and an interval $\hat{\theta} \pm 1.96 \times \text{se}(\theta) = [0.3096; 0.7344]$.

In this case, the Bayesian estimation is different from the MLE by effect of the prior information. In particular, the posterior credible interval is slightly narrower than the corresponding confidence interval, since the existing knowledge seems to be "well calibrated," i.e. in line with the observed data. Intuitively, the combination of the two consistent sources of information leads to a more precise estimation.   □

2.4.3   Monte Carlo estimation

Bayesian inference relies heavily on the computation of the posterior distribution and of some relevant syntheses. While the distribution might be known in closed form, as in the case of conjugated models, it is often not analytically tractable. At the same time, since computational power has become increasingly available in the last few years, it is sometimes easier to produce the required inference using simulation methods. Among these, one of the most important class of algorithms is represented by *Monte Carlo* (MC) methods.

The basic idea behind MC integration is that instead of performing calculation analytically, we can compute an approximate result, based on a large number of simulations from the model being investigated. The underlying assumption is that the probability distributions involved in the model are all known.

Suppose for instance that we know the functional form of the posterior distribution for the parameter of interest θ. We can draw samples from this distribution $\theta^{(1)}, \theta^{(2)}, \ldots, \theta^{(S)}$ and the mean $E(\theta)$ can be simply obtained using the MC integration instead of analytical calculations (possibly involving complex integrals) as:

$$\mathrm{E}^{MC}(\theta \mid y) = \frac{1}{S} \sum_{s=1}^{S} \theta^{(s)}.$$

Example: Modelling the number of homicides per day in London

We consider official data on the number of homicides per day observed in London in the period April 2004–March 2007, originally discussed by Spiegelhalter and Barnett (2009). Assuming that homicides occur at random, the number of murders per day can be modelled using a Poisson distribution, $y_i \mid \theta \sim \text{Poisson}(\theta)$, for $i = 1, \ldots, 1095$ days:

$$p(y_i \mid \theta) = \frac{\theta^{y_i}}{y_i!} \exp(-\theta).$$

We can assume some prior knowledge to encode the assumption that homicides are quite rare events. For example, we might assume that on average we expect less than 1 homicide per day, e.g. something between 0.25 and 0.85 murders per day. If we assume a Gamma conjugate prior $\theta \sim \text{Gamma}(\alpha_0, \beta_0)$, we can use the mathematical properties of this distribution to derive that $E(\theta) = \alpha_0/\beta_0$ and by trial and error find values of the hyper-parameters that generate a prior that is consistent with the existing information.

For example, we can use the R code[6]

```
nsim <- 1000
alpha0 <- 10
beta0 <- 20
prior <- rgamma(nsim,alpha0,beta0)
c(quantile(prior,0.025),median(prior),quantile(prior,0.975))
```

---

[6]Throughout the book, we show practical examples developed using the freely available software for statistical computing and graphics R (http://cran.r-project.org). Detailed references on how to program in R are given in Venables et al., 2011. Examples of Bayesian computations using R are also presented in Albert (2007).

which uses the built-in R function `rgamma` to generate a sample of $nsim = 1000$ simulations from a Gamma distribution with parameters $(10, 20)$.

Computing the 2.5% and the 97.5% percentiles of this vector provides an interval containing approximately 95% of the probability mass. In this case, the extremes are $(0.2617611; 0.8662637)$, which reasonably agree with the prior knowledge. Obviously, one could modify the values of (α_0, β_0) to make the prior *distribution* and the prior *information* more in line with one another. However, for the purposes of this example, we consider the prior generated by the choice $(\alpha_0, \beta_0) = (10, 20)$ as good enough.

Since the model is conjugated, it would be possible to obtain the posterior distribution in analytic form. However, it is extremely convenient to use a simulation approach and generate a sample from the posterior, which is defined according to the results shown in Table 2.3. This could be obtained by using the following code:

```
ybar <- mean(y)
alpha1 <- alpha0 + n*ybar
beta1 <- beta0 + n
posterior <- rgamma(nsim,alpha1,beta1)
```

The values stored in the vector `posterior` can be then used to produce MC summary statistics. For instance, posterior mean and variance can be computed as:

```
mean.post <- mean(posterior)
var.post <- var(posterior)
```

In the present case, the posterior mean is estimated as 0.4427, slightly lower than the prior value by effect of the observed data. In other words, on average, homicides are even rarer than we had originally thought. Moreover, approximate credible intervals can be computed by calculating the percentiles of the posterior simulations:

```
ci <- c(quantile(posterior,0.025),quantile(posterior,0.975))
```

which in this case produces the interval $[0.4055; 0.4841]$.

The precision of the MC estimation depends on the number of simulations used, as is shown in Table 2.4.

Given the simulated sample from the posterior distribution, it is easy to produce inference on relevant functions; for instance, tail area probabilities (which are sometimes referred to as "Bayesian p-values"), can be easily computed by counting the proportion of simulations exceeding a given threshold. Thus, if one were interested in estimating $\Pr(\theta > 0.5 \mid \mathbf{y})$, this would be computed as

```
p.val <- sum(posterior>0.5)/nsim
```

which in this case gives a value of 0.003.

Moreover, it is easy to sample from the predictive distribution by using the following algorithm:

TABLE 2.4

Analytical results and estimation based on MC simulations for the Poisson conjugated model

Number of simulations	MC Simulations		Analytical results
nsim	Mean	95% Credible interval	Mean
10	0.4463781	0.4074988 0.4755841	0.4421525
100	0.4384874	0.4096120 0.4781688	0.4421525
1000	0.4426710	0.4055580 0.4841028	0.4421525
10000	0.4421703	0.4044664 0.4811313	0.4421525

1. Sample a value $\theta^{(s)}$ from the posterior distribution $\theta \mid \mathbf{y} \sim \text{Gamma}(\alpha_1, \beta_1)$;

2. Sample a value $y^{*(s)}$ from a Poisson distribution with parameter $\theta^{(s)}$

3. Repeat the procedure for $s = 1, \ldots S$, where S is a large number.

In R this can be done using the following code.

```
S <- 1000
posterior <- rgamma(S,alpha1,beta1)
ystar <- rpois(S,posterior)
```

which first produces the required posterior distribution and then "mixes" it with the assumed model data. □

2.4.4 Nonconjugate priors

Since all the members of the exponential family (which includes most of the commonly used probability models) have a conjugated prior distribution, conjugacy is clearly a convenient property (Gelman et al., 2004). However, conjugated models are often too restrictive in practical modelling: they might not be flexible enough to represent available prior knowledge and for example particularly complex prior information is best encoded in the form of *mixture priors* (Robert, 2001). In addition, there are widely used models (e.g. logistic regression) for which it is not possible to identify a conjugate prior, thus limiting their usefulness in many practical applications.

Another situation where conjugacy typically does not work is when *nuisance* parameters are involved in the likelihood. For instance, suppose that we observe a vector of data $\mathbf{y}$ and are interested in a parameter θ. Suppose also that the likelihood contains an additional parameter ξ. A typical example of this situation is the case of the Normal distribution, i.e. $\mathbf{y} \sim \text{Normal}(\mu, \sigma)$. The parameters are the mean μ and the standard deviation σ, which will be typically correlated, thus implying a prior joint distribution $p(\mu, \sigma)$.

Suppose furthermore that, although we are uncertain about the actual value of σ, we are really interested only in the assessment of the mean μ. In this case, through the Bayesian approach we obtain a joint posterior distribution $p(\mu, \sigma \mid \mathbf{y})$ and we can integrate out the nuisance parameter, in order to obtain the marginal distribution of the parameter of interest:

$$p(\mu \mid \sigma, \mathbf{y}) = \int_{\mathcal{S}} p(\mu, \sigma \mid \mathbf{y}) \mathrm{d}\sigma,$$

where $\mathcal{S}$ is the domain of the variable σ, i.e. the interval $[0, \infty)$.

Unfortunately, the marginalisation process can be complex to perform in a standard form; in other words, a conjugated or analytically tractable form for the marginal posterior distribution does not always exist. Therefore approximation by simulations is the solution of choice.

Obviously, computational resources become of vital importance. In fact, the reason for the relatively limited development of Bayesian applications before the 1990s (but see Bertsch McGrayne, 2011 for some impressive counterexamples) is essentially the lack of powerful calculators able to perform the required integrations. After the great improvements in computer power, it has become relatively easy to perform Bayesian analysis with the big advantage that more complex problems can be treated. Among the simulation techniques, *Markov Chain Monte Carlo* methods play a fundamental role.

2.4.5 Markov Chain Monte Carlo methods

Markov Chain Monte Carlo (MCMC) methods are a class of algorithms for sampling from generic probability distributions — again, we do not deal here with technicalities, but refer the readers to Gilks et al. (1996), Gamerman (1997), Robert and Casella (2004), Gelman et al. (2004), Jackman (2009), Carlin and Louis (2009), Robert and Casella (2010) and Brooks et al. (2011). Robert and Casella (2011) review the history and assess the impact of MCMC.

A basic concept of MCMC methods is that of *Markov chain*, i.e. a sequence of random variables $Y_0, Y_1, Y_2, \ldots$, for which the distribution of the future state of the process, given the current and the past values, depends only on its current state:

$$p(y_{t+1} \mid y_0, y_1, \ldots, y_t) = p(y_{t+1} \mid y_t). \tag{2.16}$$

In a nutshell, MCMC methods are based on the construction of a Markov chain that converges to the desired target distribution p (i.e. the one from which we want to simulate, for instance the unknown posterior distribution of some parameter of interest). More formally, we say that p is the *stationary* distribution of the Markov chain.

Under rather broad regularity conditions which are usually met by most practical problems (Gamerman, 1997; Jackman, 2009; Brooks et al., 2011) after a sufficiently large number of iterations, referred to as *burn-in*, the chain will forget the initial state and will converge to a unique stationary distribution, which does not depend on t or Y_0. Once convergence is reached, it is possible to calculate any required statistic using MC integration.

One of the most popular MCMC methods is the *Gibbs sampling* (Geman and Geman, 1984). The main requisite to run a Gibbs sampling MCMC is that the conditional distributions of the variables of interest can be sampled from. For example, in the Bayesian context, the interest might be in the estimation of the posterior distribution of a vector of parameters $\boldsymbol{\theta} = (\theta_1, \theta_2, \ldots, \theta_K)$. The steps needed to perform an MCMC simulation via Gibbs sampling are schematically described in the following.

1. Define an initial value to be arbitrarily assigned to the parameter of interest $\theta_1^{(0)}, \theta_2^{(0)}, \ldots, \theta_K^{(0)}$.

2. Sample:

   $\theta_1^{(1)}$ from the conditional distribution $p(\theta_1 \mid \theta_2^{(0)}, \theta_3^{(0)}, \ldots, \theta_K^{(0)}, y)$;

   $\theta_2^{(1)}$ from the conditional distribution $p(\theta_2 \mid \theta_1^{(1)}, \theta_3^{(0)}, \ldots, \theta_K^{(0)}, y)$;

   $\ldots$

   $\theta_K^{(1)}$ from the conditional distribution $p(\theta_K \mid \theta_1^{(1)}, \theta_2^{(1)}, \ldots, \theta_{K-1}^{(1)}, y)$.

3. Repeat step 2. for S times until convergence is reached and produce a sample from the distribution $p(\boldsymbol{\theta} \mid y)$.

Example: Gibbs sampling for a semi-conjugated Normal model

Consider a simple model where $y_i \mid \mu, \sigma^2 \sim \text{Normal}(\theta, \sigma^2)$ for $i = 1, \ldots, n$. We assume a *semi-conjugate* prior for the parameters (Gelman et al., 2004). This entails factoring the joint prior distribution as $p(\mu, \sigma^2) = p(\mu \mid \sigma^2)p(\sigma^2)$, and then setting:

$$\mu \mid \sigma^2 \sim \text{Normal}(\mu_0, \sigma_0^2) \qquad \text{and} \qquad \tau \sim \text{Gamma}(\alpha_0, \beta_0),$$

with $\tau := 1/\sigma^2$ indicating the *precision* of the Normal distribution.

This model encodes three fundamental assumptions:

A1. the two components of the parameter vector $\boldsymbol{\theta} = (\mu, \sigma^2)$ are considered *independent a priori*; this might be a reasonable assumption when uncertainty about the mean is assessed with no reference to prior measurements characterised by a variance σ^2;

A2. conditionally on the value of σ^2, the prior distribution for μ is conjugated with the data model;

A3. similarly, the marginal prior distribution for the precision τ is conjugated.

Notice that the joint prior distribution is not conjugate for the Normal likelihood. In fact, μ and σ^2 are dependent in the resulting posterior. However, in order to estimate the posterior distribution of $\boldsymbol{\theta}$ using the Gibbs sampling, we only need the *full conditional* distributions $p(\mu \mid \sigma^2, \mathbf{y})$ and $p(\sigma^2 \mid \mu, \mathbf{y})$.

Because of A2. and A3. the relevant conditional distributions are conjugated and therefore:

$$p(\mu \mid \tau, \mathbf{y}) = \text{Normal}(\mu_n, \sigma_n^2)$$

$$= \text{Normal}\left(\frac{\frac{\mu_0}{\sigma_0^2} + \frac{n\bar{y}}{\sigma^2}}{\frac{1}{\sigma_0^2} + \frac{n}{\sigma^2}}, \frac{1}{\frac{1}{\sigma_0^2} + \frac{n}{\sigma^2}}\right) \qquad (2.17)$$

and

$$p(\tau \mid \mu, \mathbf{y}) = \text{Gamma}(\alpha_n, \beta_n)$$

$$= \text{Gamma}\left(\alpha_0 + \frac{n}{2}, \beta_0 + \frac{\sum_{i=1}^{n}(y_i - \mu)^2}{2}\right) \qquad (2.18)$$

(cfr. the analysis of Table 2.3).

Suppose that we observe a sample of $n = 30$ data points $\mathbf{y}$:

$y_1 = 1.2697$	$y_2 = 7.7637$	$y_3 = 2.2532$	$y_4 = 3.4557$	$y_5 = 4.1776$
$y_6 = 6.4320$	$y_7 = -3.6623$	$y_8 = 7.7567$	$y_9 = 5.9032$	$y_{10} = 7.2671$
$y_{11} = -2.3447$	$y_{12} = 8.0160$	$y_{13} = 3.5013$	$y_{14} = 2.8495$	$y_{15} = 0.6467$
$y_{16} = 3.2371$	$y_{17} = 5.8573$	$y_{18} = -3.3749$	$y_{19} = 4.1507$	$y_{20} = 4.3092$
$y_{21} = 11.7327$	$y_{22} = 2.6174$	$y_{23} = 9.4942$	$y_{24} = -2.7639$	$y_{25} = -1.5859$
$y_{26} = 3.6986$	$y_{27} = 2.4544$	$y_{28} = -0.3294$	$y_{29} = 0.2329$	$y_{30} = 5.2846$

which give a sample mean $\bar{y} = 3.3433$. We complete the model by specifying values of the hyper-parameters to obtain minimally informative priors, for instance $\mu_0 = 0, \sigma_0^2 = 10\,000, \alpha_0 = 0.01$ and $\beta_0 = 0.01$).

The following R code[7] programs the required Gibbs sampling.

```
# Loads the data
y <- c(1.2697,7.7637,2.2532,3.4557,4.1776,6.4320,-3.6623,7.7567,
       5.9032,7.2671,-2.3447,8.0160,3.5013,2.8495,0.6467,3.2371,
       5.8573,-3.3749,4.1507,4.3092,11.7327,2.6174,9.4942,-2.7639,
       -1.5859,3.6986,2.4544,-0.3294,0.2329,5.2846)
ybar <- mean(y)
n <- length(y)

# Defines the hyper-parameters to build the full conditionals
mu_0 <- 0
sigma2_0 <- 10000
alpha_0 <- 0.01
beta_0 <- 0.01

# Initialises the parameters selecting a random starting point
mu <- tau <- numeric()
sigma2 <- 1/tau
mu[1] <- rnorm(1,0,5)
tau[1] <- runif(1,0,5)
```

---

[7]The computer codes and some of the datasets discussed throughout the book can be downloaded at www.statistca.it/gianluca/BMHE.

```
sigma2[1] <- 1/tau[1]

# Gibbs sampling (samples from the full conditionals)
nsim <- 1000
for (i in 2:nsim) {
    sigma2_n <- 1/(1/sigma2_0 + n/sigma2[i-1])
    mu_n <- (mu_0/sigma2_0 + n*ybar/sigma2[i-1])/sigma2_n
    mu[i] <- rnorm(1,mu_n,sqrt(sigma2_n))

    alpha_n <- alpha_0+n/2
    beta_n <- beta_0 + sum((y-mu[i])^2)/2
    tau[i] <- rgamma(1,alpha_n,beta_n)
    sigma2[i] <- 1/tau[i]
}
```

First, the data are loaded into R in the vector y. Then the hyper-parameters are defined and the vectors mu and tau are created and initialised using random starting points. Alternatively, we could have set mu[1] and tau[1] to some fixed values. Then, we iteratively sample from the full conditional distributions (2.17) and (2.18) for a large number nsim of times. At each iteration, the hyper-parameters are updated. In particular, first we update the mean mu[i] using the *current* value of the variance sigma2[i-1]. Then we update the variance using the value of the mean that we have just simulated.

Figure 2.10 shows the Gibbs sampling simulation at different numbers of iterations. While the first few iterations can visit peripheral points (depending also on the initial values), because of conditional conjugacy, already after 30 iterations the procedure seems to concentrate on points that lie in the relevant area of the posterior density. Notice that the graph shows the joint distribution of (μ, σ), but given the simulations for the variance, it is easy to compute sigma <- sqrt(sigma2).

Using the vector of simulations, it is possible to compute the posterior summaries for the parameters. The posterior mean for μ is 2.10 and a 95% credible interval is computed as $[-1.27; 5.40]$. Similar statistics for the standard deviation σ are 9.27 and $[7.08; 12.34]$. □

2.4.6 MCMC convergence

The main properties of an MCMC analysis, which need to be evaluated carefully before any inference can be drawn from it, are *convergence* and *autocorrelation*. An MCMC run is in general dependent on the initial values selected for the chains and the first few iterations typically provide values that do not have high probability under that distribution. Consequently, to make an inference based (also) on these values will invariably produce a bias in the results. For this reason, it is fundamental to assess convergence and to discard the burn-in iterations before producing the required estimations.

Figure 2.11 shows intuitively the concept of convergence of a Markov chain; in order to evaluate actual convergence, we typically run several parallel

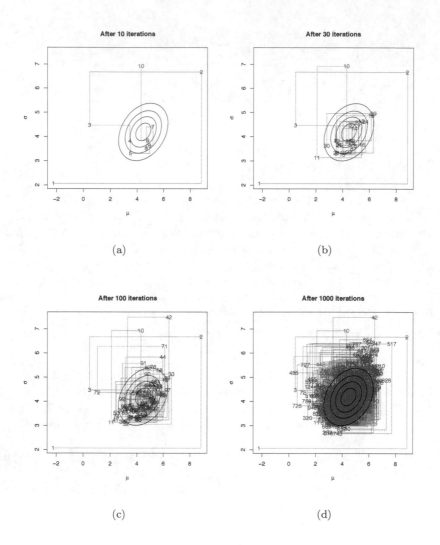

FIGURE 2.10
Gibbs sampling simulation for the semi-conjugated Normal model. The numbers indicate the simulations sequence. Panels (a)–(d) show the situation after 10, 30, 100 and 1000 iterations respectively. In this case, already 100, or even 30 simulations seem to cover the relevant portion of the parametric space.

chains, for which we set quite different starting points. Initially, the sampled values depend on the initial points and will tend to visit areas of the target space that might be quite far from the main probability mass. However, after a period of burn-in, the chains will tend to converge to the target distribution.

This process is often referred to as "mixing-up." Once this happens, we typically discard the pre-convergence simulations and base the MC estimation on the post-convergence sample.

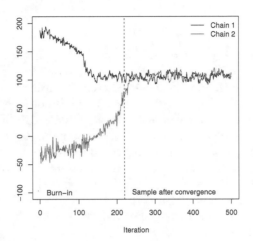

FIGURE 2.11

Graphical assessment of convergence for a Markov chain; in this case two chains are set up, starting from different initial points. After the burn-in period, the two chains converge to the stationary distribution.

The most used formal method to assess convergence is the Gelman and Rubin (1992) statistic. The main idea is that two or more chains should be run and started from different initial values, which should be chosen to have larger variance than the one thought to underlie the data, while still being "reasonable" points. Given the output from the multiple MCMC runs, convergence can be assessed by comparing the between-chains to the within-chain variation for each scalar component of the vector of parameters of interest.

Thus, if the parameters are $\boldsymbol{\theta} = (\theta_1, \ldots, \theta_K)$, the posterior variance of the generic component θ_k can be estimated as:

$$\widehat{\mathrm{Var}}(\theta_k \mid \mathbf{y}) = \frac{S-1}{S} W(\theta_k) + \frac{1}{S} B(\theta_k),$$

where $W(\theta_k)$ and $B(\theta_k)$ are the average within-chain variance and the between-chains variance, and S is the length of the MCMC sample. Convergence is then monitored by assessing the *potential scale reduction*

$$\hat{R} = \sqrt{\frac{\widehat{\mathrm{Var}}(\theta_k \mid \mathbf{y})}{W(\theta_k)}}, \tag{2.19}$$

which represents the factor by which the scale of the current estimated posterior distribution of θ_k can be further reduced. If $\hat{R}$ is large, then considering a longer MCMC run will potentially improve the inference about the target distribution. As a rule of thumb, values of $\hat{R} \leq 1.1$ are generally accepted as indicative of sufficient convergence.

2.4.7   MCMC autocorrelation

The second critical aspect of MCMC procedures is that the iterations produced by a Markov chain are by definition correlated, since the current observation depends on the previous one. Therefore, intuitively the actual number of iterations stored to produce the inference does not give in general the same information provided by a sample of *iid* observations of the same size. In other words, the higher the autocorrelation, the lower the degree of equivalence between the MCMC output and a proper *iid* sample of the same size.

For this reason, it is useful to assess the number of equivalent independent observations that are associated with the actual sample of values generated by the MCMC run. In simple terms, the lower the decay of autocorrelation with the increased number of simulations used, the smaller the *effective sample size* n_{eff}. In particular, it holds that:

$$n_{\text{eff}} = \frac{S}{1 + 2\sum_{t=1}^{\infty} \rho_t}, \tag{2.20}$$

where ρ_t is the lag t autocorrelation (i.e. the correlation between two iterations that are t time steps apart) for a given parameter. Thus, when n_{eff} is close to S, the level of autocorrelation is negligible and convergence is reasonably reached.

Notice that, even in the presence of autocorrelation, convergence might still be reached (as confirmed by the value of the Gelman–Rubin statistics). However, the increased level of autocorrelation makes the estimation of the entire posterior distribution less precise. In particular, when n_{eff} is much smaller than the actual number of iterations simulated, then the extreme quantiles of the posterior distribution are typically estimated without precision (Jackman, 2009).

An alternative way of decreasing autocorrelation is to *thin* the chains, i.e. to run the MCMC algorithm for S iterations while monitoring only one every t. This is reasonable because usually autocorrelation decreases at higher lags. Obviously, thinning means that to produce inference based on H simulations, it is necessary to run a single chain for Ht iterations, or more generally, if c chains are run simultaneously, for Ht/c times.

Alternative procedures to the Gibbs sampling have been recently investigated, e.g. Integrated Nested Laplace Approximation (INLA, Rue et al, 2009) and Hamiltonian Monte Carlo (Girolami and Calderhead, 2011), which can reduce the computation time and limit convergence problems, especially for non-Normal, complex models. Such methods can be helpful in the analysis of hierarchical models (cfr. §5.3).

Example: Checking and improving convergence of the Gibbs sampling

One of the easiest ways to improve convergence is to break the correlation between the variables to be estimated. The simplest example occurs in linear regression analysis with observed data $y_i \sim \text{Normal}(\mu_i, \sigma^2)$ for $i = 1, \ldots, N$.

First we consider one possible model, say $\mathcal{M}_1$, which assumes $\mu_i = \alpha + \beta X_i$ with simple minimally informative prior distributions on the regression coefficients $\alpha, \beta \sim \text{Normal}(0, 10000)$ independently, and on the logarithm of the standard deviation $\log(\sigma) \sim \text{Uniform}(-k, k)$, for a large value k. Then, we build a second model $\mathcal{M}_2$ in which $\mu_i = \alpha + \beta Z_i$ and $Z_i = X_i - \bar{X}$, i.e. we *centre* the covariate X around its mean, and the same prior distributions for α, β and $\log(\sigma)$.

The two models differ only in the way that the covariate X is specified, but the definition of the prior distributions is unchanged. In fact, in this simple case, the posterior distributions could be derived analytically (Gelman et al., 2004), but can also be simulated using Gibbs sampling.

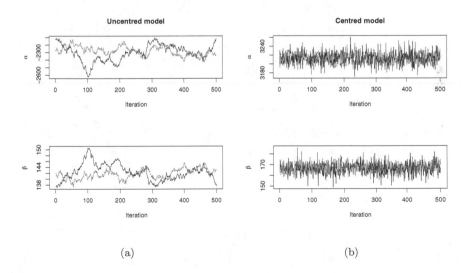

(a)   (b)

FIGURE 2.12
Traceplots for the parameters (α, β): in model $\mathcal{M}_1$ (a) the mixing of the two chains is poor, so that convergence is not reached. In Model $\mathcal{M}_2$ (b), the two chains are consistently visiting the same portion of the parametric space, which is indication of convergence of the Gibbs sampling.

Figure 2.12 shows the traceplots for 500 iterations (monitored after a burn in of 9500 runs for two chains) from the posterior distribution of the regression coefficients for model. In particular, Figures 2.12(a) and (b) show the results for models $\mathcal{M}_1$ and $\mathcal{M}_2$ respectively. As one can see, it is obvious even just looking at the traceplots that the mixing of the model with uncentred covariate is not good enough. On the contrary, with the same number of iterations and using exactly the same specifications for the priors, model $\mathcal{M}_2$ has reached a quite satisfactory level of mixing up between the two chains.

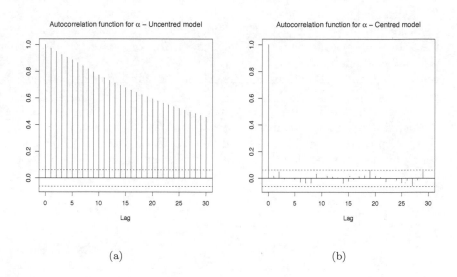

(a)   (b)

FIGURE 2.13
Autocorrelation function for the parameter α. In the uncentred model (a), autocorrelation is quite high and remains so even at high lags. The centred model (b), on the other hand, shows extremely low levels of autocorrelation among the iterations even at low lags.

Figure 2.13(a) confirms the poor mixing of model $\mathcal{M}_1$ by showing the autocorrelation function (correlogram) for the parameter α. Even for high lags, autocorrelation remains high, whereas in model $\mathcal{M}_2$, the situation is reversed and the simulations do not show high levels of autocorrelation even at low lags — cfr. Figure 2.13(b).

The reason why the uncentred model has more problems in converging and exploring the relevant space is shown in Figure 2.14(a). The regression coefficients (α, β) have a very large correlation (in fact, the correlation between the posterior simulations is -0.988). On the contrary, as shown in Figure 2.14(b), centering X around its mean in model $\mathcal{M}_2$ has the effect of breaking up the correlation between the parameters bringing it to an observed level of -0.038.

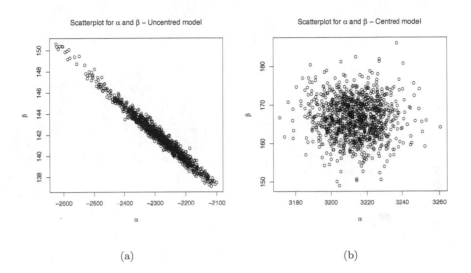

(a) (b)

FIGURE 2.14

Scatterplot for the regression coefficients (α, β) for the uncentred (a) and the centred (b) models. Centering the covariate X has the effect of breaking up the correlation between the two parameters, thus improving convergence.

Intuitively, this helps convergence because with lower correlation the joint posterior of the parameters has a more disperse shape. Thus, even lengthy moves from one iteration to the next visit relevant parts of the density. On the contrary, a joint posterior distribution that is characterised by large correlation has a much narrower shape (cfr. Figure 2.14), which means that a large number of small moves are required to cover all the relevant part of the parametric space.

An alternative to centering X is to use "brute force" and run model $\mathcal{M}_1$ for a very large number of iterations, possibly thinning the chains. We performed a Gibbs sampling run of 50000 iterations using a burn-in of 9500 and then a thinning of 81 simulations (i.e. one in every 81 of the 40500 iterations obtained is monitored and used to perform the analysis). The mixing of the chains is very much improved, and in fact the traceplot of Figure 2.15(a) gives an indication of convergence. The correlogram for alpha shows that there is still some autocorrelation present, but to a much lower extent than in the previous case.

Incidentally, in the uncentred model, $\hat{R} = 1.145$ for α and 1.140 for β, while $n_{\text{eff}} = 37$ and 38, respectively (as opposed to $500 \times 2 = 1000$ iterations

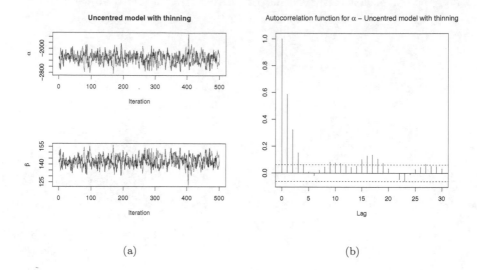

(a)   (b)

FIGURE 2.15

Traceplot for the regression coefficients of model $\mathcal{M}_1$ using 50000 iterations with a burn-in of 9500 and thinning of 81 (a); Autocorrelation function for the parameter α (b). The traceplot especially indicates that convergence is now reached.

actually monitored). When thinning is applied to a longer run, $\hat{R} = 1.007$ for both α and β, and $n_{\text{eff}} = 370$. Similarly, for $\mathcal{M}_2$ $\hat{R} = 1.004$ for α and 1.005 for β, and $n_{\text{eff}} = 370$ and 320, respectively.

Alternative methods to improve convergence by breaking up correlation among the parameters in more complex situations (for example by means of redundant parameterisations) are discussed at length in Gelman et al. (2004), Gelman and Hill (2007) and Jackman (2009).

In any case, the current example shows the importance of carefully monitoring the convergence and mixing up the chains. To this aim, the best strategy probably includes a combination of formal (such as the analysis of the $\hat{R}$ statistic) and informal methods, including traceplots and autocorrelation graphs. Additional statistics, such as Raftery–Lewis diagnostic (Raftery and Lewis, 1995) can be used to investigate the accuracy of the estimation for a given quantile of the posterior distribution of interest (cfr. §4.3.4).   □

As appears clear from the previous examples, programming a Gibbs sampling run is actually quite easy when the full conditional distributions are known analytically. Unfortunately, this does not necessarily happen and in fact in the large majority of cases one needs to resort to simulation strategies just because the form of the relevant distributions is not known or tractable.

However, it is possible to complement the simple structure of a Gibbs sampling program with other well established algorithms in a two-step procedure. First, we use a specialised algorithm, as for instance Metropolis-Hastings (Metropolis et al., 1953; Hastings, 1970) or the slice sampling (Neal, 2003), to provide a reasonable approximation to the required unknown conditional distribution. Then, Gibbs sampling is implemented using this approximation to derive the required target. This effectively allows one to sample from virtually any posterior distribution.

In particular, general purpose samplers such as WinBUGS (Spiegelhalter et al., 2002) or JAGS (Plummer, 2010) have been developed in the last twenty years, which are able to apply the most effective combination of sampling algorithms to perform Gibbs sampling of a given model. Chapter 4 is focussed on the application of Bayesian models using these particular pieces of software.

3

Statistical cost-effectiveness analysis

3.1 Introduction

In the last ten years, health economic evaluations have built on more advanced statistical decision-theoretic foundations, effectively becoming a branch of applied statistics (Briggs et al., 2006; Willan and Briggs, 2006), increasingly often under a Bayesian statistical approach (O'Hagan and Stevens, 2001; O'Hagan et al., 2001; Parmigiani, 2002b; Spiegelhalter and Best, 2003; Spiegelhalter et al., 2004).

As suggested by Spiegelhalter et al. (2004), this can be ascribed to the fact that "the subjective interpretation of probability is essential, since the expressions of uncertainty required for a decision analysis can rarely be based purely on empirical data."

Even though the process is, technically, a simple application of standard decision-theoretic precepts (described for example in Lindley, 1985), health economics is complicated by issues related to other important factors that play a major role in real practice medical decision making. Among these are the difficulty of applying standard cost-effectiveness techniques to the regulatory process (Baio and Russo, 2009), and the necessity of properly accounting for the impact of uncertainty in the inputs of decision processes, an issue known as *sensitivity analysis* (Parmigiani, 2002b; Saltelli et al., 2004). This latter in particular is fundamental and is a required basic component of any new drug approval or reimbursement dossier in settings regulated by decision-making bodies such as NICE in the UK (Claxton et al., 2005).

In this chapter we first briefly review the main characteristics of decision theory. As in Chapter 2 we proceed by introducing the more abstract theory, in order to make the point that rational decision-making is effected by maximising the expectation of a suitably defined utility function. This is used to quantify the value associated with the uncertain consequences of a possible intervention.

Next we link the general methodology to the specific problem faced in health economic evaluation. This requires the specification of the problem in terms of a composite response, accounting for both cost and benefits. We present a relatively simple running example and, as in Chapter 2, we switch between the development of the theory and its application throughout.

We then concentrate on the development of sensitivity analysis techniques, which as suggested earlier, play a fundamental role in health economic evaluations. Finally, we present some more advanced issues associated with the main assumptions on which cost-effectiveness or cost-utility analyses are based: in particular, we consider the problems of risk-aversion and the impact of market constraints (e.g. in the case of regulatory processes).

3.2 Decision theory and expected utility

3.2.1 Problem

Health economic evaluations are a typical problem of decision-making under uncertainty. The main objective is to evaluate comparatively the unknown consequences of a given health intervention against at least another. A suitable approach to deal with this kind of problems is based on *expected utility theory*, which we briefly review in this section. More substantial references are Savage (1954), Raiffa (1968), Lindley (1985), Berger (1985), Smith (1988), Bernardo and Smith (1999), Parmigiani (2002b), Jordaan (2005) and Smith (2011).

Formally, a decision problem is characterised by some fundamental elements: first, we consider the possible *decisions* (interventions, actions, treatments) $t \in \mathcal{T}$, representing the alternatives available to the decision-maker. The selection of each possible intervention has some *consequences* (outcomes) $o \in \mathcal{O}$, defined in general as functions of suitable random quantities $\boldsymbol{\omega} \in \Omega$. Every consequence can be expressed as $o = (\boldsymbol{\omega}, t)$, i.e. as the result of choosing intervention t and the fact that a series of random quantities $\boldsymbol{\omega}$ will obtain in the future. The set of consequences can be then represented as $\mathcal{O} = \Omega \times \mathcal{T}$.

In addition to these fundamental quantities, the decision-maker needs to define a scheme of *preferences* among the many decisions and consequences; this relationship of preference is generically indicated by the symbol '$\preceq$'. The notation $t_1 \preceq t_2$ indicates that the random consequences of action t_1 are *not* preferred to those of action t_2. If $t_1 \preceq t_2$ and simultaneously $t_2 \preceq t_1$, the two actions are indifferent: $t_1 \sim t_2$.

The Bayesian decision process is based on a set of *prescriptive axioms*. These are the criteria that *should* hold in order to make rational decisions. The first set of axioms is related to the *coherence* of the decision making and involves:

- *comparability of the consequences*. This assumes that the decision-maker is capable of producing some form of ranking of the possible outcomes, so that there exist at least one pair of consequences o_1 and o_2 for which the former is preferred to the latter;

- *transitivity of the preferences*. This axiom implies that if the decision-maker has a preference for action t_2 over action t_1 and for action t_3 over action t_2, then $t_1 \preceq t_3$. The intuition behind this axiom is that if transitivity did not hold (e.g. the case where $t_1 \preceq t_2$, $t_2 \preceq t_3$ and $t_3 \preceq t_1$), sequential decision-making could lead to very strange behaviour. For example, a decision-maker faced with the choice between the actions t_1 and t_2 would select the latter, perhaps at a cost c_{12}; similarly, when comparing t_2 and t_3, the decision-maker should choose the latter (this time at a cost of say c_{23}). But when comparing t_1 and t_3, if transitivity did not hold, the decision-maker would select t_1 (say at a cost c_{13}), thus going back to precisely the same position they were at the beginning, but having paid $c_{12} + c_{23} + c_{31}$ in the process;

- *consistency of the preferences.* This axiom codifies the intuition that if a decision-maker prefers an action to another when certain events occur, but also when these events do not occur, then the choice is void and the action is always preferred. In other words, in a similar situation, uncertainty is effectively irrelevant ("sure thing principle," Savage, 1954).

The second set of axioms is more technical and codifies *quantifiability*, i.e. the existence of standard reference events and measurement of the preferences.

If the decision-maker behaves in such a way that these axioms are verified, then the rationality of the decision process is guaranteed (cfr. §2.2.3). In particular, in order to proceed rationally in the analysis of the decision process under uncertainty, Bayesian decision theory (de Finetti, 1974; Bernardo and Smith, 1999) prescribes that:

- uncertainty about the random quantities is quantified using a suitable subjective *probability measure* $p(\boldsymbol{\omega})$, i.e. a function $p : \Omega \to [0; 1]$ associating a number in $[0, 1]$ with each random quantity that is relevant for the problem at hand;

- the value of each outcome is quantified by means of a *measure of utility* $u : \mathcal{O} \to \mathbb{R}$, of the form $u(o) = u(\boldsymbol{\omega}, t)$, i.e. a function associating a real number to the set of consequences. This can be constructed, for example, using the standard gamble technique (cfr. §1.4.3).

In general, the relevant random quantities in a decision problem can be partitioned as $\boldsymbol{\omega} = (y, \boldsymbol{\theta})$. Here $y \in \mathcal{Y}$ indicates the observable *future results* for an individual or group of individuals, conditionally on the application of a given intervention t. With $\boldsymbol{\theta} \in \Theta$ we identify a set of *parameters*, characterising the probability distribution of y. On the basis of this assumption, it is possible to express $p(\boldsymbol{\omega}) = p(y, \boldsymbol{\theta}) = p(y \mid \boldsymbol{\theta})p(\boldsymbol{\theta})$, in line with the Bayesian approach described in Chapter 2.

A further assumption that is usually reasonable is that the consequences of the decision-maker's actions depend directly only on y, i.e. the future results experienced by the individuals. On the contrary, the parameters $\boldsymbol{\theta}$ are only indirectly relevant to the inferential process described by the probability distribution $p(y \mid \boldsymbol{\theta})$. Consequently, the outcomes are indicated as $o = (y, t)$ and the utility function associated with them is $u(y, t)$.

3.2.2   Decision criterion: Maximisation of the expected utility

The final aspect of a decision problem is concerned with the definition of a suitable rule that allows the decision-maker to select the "optimal" strategy (intervention). One obvious criterion to assess and compare a set of available interventions is to select the one associated with the highest chance of obtaining the preferred consequence.

The remarkable result of decision theory is that, because of the way in which the utility measure is defined (e.g. by means of the standard gamble procedure), in order to maximise the chance of obtaining the preferred outcome, it suffices to maximise the expectation of the utility measure, since the two can be proved to be equivalent. Thus, decision making can be effected by simply computing an average, rather than dealing with probabilities.

Example: Expected utility as the probability of obtaining the preferred outcome

Suppose that the interest is in a disease characterised by a subset of S states among those identified by the SF-6D, for which a valuation in terms of utility scores exist (e.g. as in Table 1.2). For the sake of simplicity, we assume that two interventions are available to treat the disease, i.e. $\mathcal{T} = (0,1)$, and that the relevant $S = 5$ health states are $y_1 = 111111$ (perfect health, which is obviously the preferred outcome), $y_2 = 111122$, $y_3 = 433433$, $y_4 = 645655$ and $y_5 =$ death (which we assume to be the least favourite outcome).

For each individual in the population of interest, we can define a vector of parameters $\boldsymbol{\theta}^t$, whose elements θ_s^t indicate the probability that state $s = 1, \ldots, S$ will obtain if intervention t is applied. In order to prove the point without unnecessary mathematical complications, for the moment we unrealistically assume that these probabilities are known without uncertainty.

Under these assumptions, the preferred outcome of perfect health can be obtained in either of the two following cases:

- *directly*, which under each intervention occurs with probability θ_1^t;

- *virtually* (or indirectly), when any other state obtains (each with the associated probability of θ_s^t). In fact, any other state y_s is by definition of the utilities equivalent to a scenario in which perfect health is obtained with probability $\pi_s = u(y_s, t)$.

Thus, because the two cases above are by definition mutually exclusive (i.e. they cannot both happen at the same time), by the law of total probability the chance of obtaining the preferred consequence y_1 (i.e. the state of perfect health) is

$$
\begin{aligned}
\Pr(y_1 \mid \boldsymbol{\theta}^t) &= \theta_1^t + \sum_{s=2}^{S} \pi_s \times \Pr(y_s \mid \boldsymbol{\theta}^t) \\
&= \sum_{s=1}^{S} \pi_s \times \theta_s^t \\
&= \sum_{s=1}^{S} u(y_s, t) \times \theta_s^t \\
&= \mathrm{E}\left[u(Y, t)\right],
\end{aligned}
\tag{3.1}
$$

since by definition $\pi_1 = u(y_1, t) = 1$ and $\theta_s^t = \Pr(y_s \mid \boldsymbol{\theta}^t)$.

Moreover, it is possible to prove that in general there exist two values $a > 0$ and b such that another utility function $u^*(y, t) = au(y, t) + b$ exists, which describes the same scheme of preference as the original one $u(y, t)$. This allows us to generalise the definition of the utility function (Robert, 2001). $\square$

As suggested above, the implication of (3.1) is that the probability of obtaining the preferred option is equivalent to the the expected value of the utility function, more commonly referred to as the *expected utility*. We indicate this quantity with the symbol $\mathcal{U}^t$.

Therefore, on the basis of the assumption of coherence in the comparison among random events and consequences, *the optimal decision criterion is the maximisation of the expected utility*. This is effectively equivalent to maximising the probability of occurrence of the preferred outcome. The optimal action which should be selected by the decision-maker is then

$$
t^* = \arg\max_{\mathcal{T}} \mathcal{U}^t.
$$

This result is rather important, as it provides a unique criterion to rank the many available options, on the basis of the available information.

Of course, in general it is not possible to know the value of the parameters without uncertainty and therefore within a Bayesian framework it will be necessary to model them using a suitable distribution $p(\boldsymbol{\theta}^t \mid \mathcal{D})$, conditionally on the background information $\mathcal{D}$. Moreover, the individual response might be characterised by a continuous random variable, rather than a discrete set of states, as in (3.1). Although the interpretation remains the same, in this more general case the expected utility is expressed as

$$
\mathcal{U}^t = \int \int u(y, t)\, p(y \mid \boldsymbol{\theta}^t)\, p(\boldsymbol{\theta}^t \mid \mathcal{D})\, \mathrm{d}y\, \mathrm{d}\boldsymbol{\theta}^t,
\tag{3.2}
$$

and is obtained by averaging over the uncertainty in both *population* ("objective") and *parameters* ("subjective") domains.

Notice that while the utility *function* $u(y, t)$ associates a real number with the set of outcomes $\mathcal{O} = \Omega \times \mathcal{T}$, the *expected* utility $\mathcal{U} : \mathcal{T} \to \mathbb{R}$ associates a unique numerical value with each option t. This is consistent with the marginalisation process operated on the uncertainty about the random quantities on Ω.

As remarked by Spiegelhalter et al. (2004), the frequentist version of decision theory does not produce an average with respect to prior or posterior distributions. Thus, the decision-making strategy generally maximises the utility, whatever the "true" value of the parameter might be. This can be thought of as assuming the most pessimistic prior distribution.

The Bayesian procedure can be then seen as a generalisation of the frequentist analysis, with the usual advantage of explicitly accounting for all forms of recognised uncertainty (both on the "individual" and "population" levels).

3.3   Decision-making in health economics

In a typical health economic problem, we are interested in the management of a particular clinical condition for which a set of interventions $t \in \mathcal{T} = (0, 1, \ldots, T-1)$ is available. We can apply a generic intervention t to any unit i in the relevant population and observe a (possibly multivariate) response, y_i. Typically, y_i will be represented by a suitable clinical outcome (e.g. blood pressure or occurrence of myocardial infarction), together with a measure of the costs associated with the given intervention. In general, we then write $y = (e, c)$.

The objective of the health economic evaluation is to decide which treatment to apply to a new unit i', judged as similar to, or, in statistical terms, exchangeable (cfr. §2.3.1) with all the others receiving the same treatment. In particular, we take the standpoint of a body that is responsible for issuing guidance on the implementation of alternative interventions for specific public health matters. As suggested earlier, a standard programme will be typically available and a new one is suggested to replace it, perhaps partially or only on specific sub-populations of individuals. The argument can easily be extended to $T > 2$ different treatments; however, for the sake of simplicity we here confine attention to the case $\mathcal{T} = (0, 1)$.

Example: Modelling the cost-effectiveness of a new chemotherapy drug

Suppose the interest is in evaluating a new chemotherapy drug for the treatment of cancer against the standard one. After the drug is administered, patients may or may not show some haematological (blood related) side effects.

If this does happen, depending on the gravity of the side effects, patients either need ambulatory care or are admitted to hospital.

The focus is on the clinical and economic evaluation of the policy that makes the new drug available ($t = 1$) against the null option ($t = 0$) under which the standard drug is used. A detailed description of the programming aspects related with this model is presented in §4.7 □

3.3.1 Statistical framework

The assumption of exchangeability essentially amounts to assuming the following data-generating process for the observables y_i (Baio and Dawid, 2011). First, we introduce a population parameter $\boldsymbol{\theta}$, generally involving treatment specific components: $\boldsymbol{\theta} = (\theta^0, \theta^1)$. The current *uncertainty* about $\boldsymbol{\theta}$ is formally described by a suitable probability distribution. This is computed starting from a (possibly subjective) prior distribution that describes the state of science about the parameters before observing any new data. For example, for each possible intervention t, patient-level data may be available (as produced by a set of randomised trials or observational studies) in the form $\mathcal{D}^t = \{y_i : i = 1, \ldots, n_t\}$. We generally refer to the whole set of background information as $\mathcal{D} = \bigcup_t \mathcal{D}^t$. The joint distribution of all the parameters is then $p(\boldsymbol{\theta} \mid \mathcal{D})$, from which it is possible to obtain every single marginal distribution $p(\theta^t \mid \mathcal{D})$.

Conditionally on $\boldsymbol{\theta}$ and a proposed treatment t, the second step of the data generation process consists of drawing the y_i's independently from the probability distribution $p(y \mid \theta^t)$, which describes the individual *variability* of the future (yet unobserved) health economic response. A similar general framework has been described in the health economic literature by O'Hagan and Stevens (2001) and Parmigiani (2002b).

Example (continued)

We describe here the model used for the chemotherapy drug problem. We indicate with π_t the probability that a patient selected at random from the relevant population and treated with drug $t = 0, 1$ (to indicate the standard or the new drug, respectively) shows blood related side effects after treatment.

More specifically, perhaps following preliminary data obtained by randomised studies performed by the company that are seeking to market the new option, we assume that $\pi_1 = \pi_0 \rho$, where ρ represents the reduction in the occurrence of side effects generated by the new drug. This implies that π_0 and π_1 are correlated.

Conditionally on π_t, we indicate the probability of needing ambulatory care as γ. Then, given the simple structure of our model, the probability that a patient showing side effects requires hospital admission is set to $(1 - \gamma)$. Note that, in general, this might be an unrealistic assumption, as other interventions might be required to deal with side effects (e.g. additional drug therapies). However, for the sake of simplicity, we assume that this is a reasonable representation of the clinical problem under study.

With these assumptions and setting the total number of patients in the reference population to $N = 1\,000$, we can also define the number of patients experiencing side effects as $SE_t \sim \text{Binomial}(\pi_t, N)$; the total number of patients with side effects requiring ambulatory care as $A_t \sim \text{Binomial}(\gamma, SE_t)$; and the total number of patients with side effects requiring hospital admission as $H_t = SE_t - A_t$.

As for the costs, we consider a fixed value to represent the cost of acquisition of the two drugs, which we indicate by c_t^{drug}. All patients are subjected to this cost. However, depending on whether or not they experience side effects, there are possible additional costs, represented by c^{amb} (for ambulatory care) and c^{hosp} (hospital admission). It is reasonable to assume that these two costs are independent of the treatment being administered.

With respect to the discussion of §3.3.1, the assumptions encoded by this model are that we consider a population parameter $\boldsymbol{\theta} = (\boldsymbol{\theta}^0, \boldsymbol{\theta}^1)$, with the two components being defined as $\boldsymbol{\theta}^0 = (\pi_0, \gamma, c^{\text{amb}}, c^{\text{hosp}})$ and $\boldsymbol{\theta}^1 = (\pi_1, \gamma, c^{\text{amb}}, c^{\text{hosp}})$.

We assume that the existing evidence comprises 5 small studies performed under the standard treatment on the number of patients experiencing side effects and those among them requiring ambulatory care. Therefore, we assume conjugate minimally informative priors (cfr. §2.4.1) for the parameters π_0 and γ and use this evidence to inform their posterior.

For the remaining parameters in $\boldsymbol{\theta}$, we assume informative prior distributions as specified in Table 3.1, which are derived by using suitable hyper-parameters that have been set to encode knowledge $\mathcal{D}$ available from previous studies and expert opinion.

For example, a Normal distribution with hyper-parameters $\mu = 0.8$ and $\sigma = 0.2$ has the property of having a mean value of 0.8 and contains 95% of the probability mass in the interval $[0.40 - 1.20]$. This is taken to be consistent with what is suggested by the limited evidence and the theory underlying the reduction in the chance of side effects for patients treated with the innovative chemotherapy drug. It is therefore possible to encode the prior knowledge on ρ using such a simple distributional assumption.

Notice however that, because ρ is a relative risk, it is defined to be positive and may present some skewness. Thus an alternative specification of the prior that would better account for these characteristics would be for example in the form $\log(\rho) \sim \text{Normal}(\mu, \sigma)$. In this case, the hyper-parameters (μ, σ) would be defined on the log scale (we return to this issues with more details in Chapters 4 and 5).

As discussed at length in §2.4, the choice of the prior distributions is a matter of context knowledge; for instance, parameters representing the probability of occurrence of an event, e.g. the chance of having ambulatory care following side effects *can* (but do not necessarily *have to*) be modelled by using a Beta distribution. This is just a mathematical convenience, and in fact it is

TABLE 3.1

Distributional assumptions for the model. For each parameter, the distributions are chosen to model the available prior knowledge, represented by existing data or expert opinions. The mathematical form of the distributions is chosen according to the nature of the parameter (i.e. parameters describing probability of occurrence of an event are usually given a Beta distribution), while the values of the hyper-parameters are chosen so that the distribution is consistent with the prior information derived by the clinical literature or expert opinion.

	Mean	2.5%	Median	97.5%	Distribution
π_0	0.500	0.0017	0.4990	0.9986	Beta(0.5, 0.5)
ρ	0.8004	0.4058	0.7913	1.1702	Normal(0.8, 0.2)
γ	0.500	0.0017	0.4990	0.9986	Beta(0.5, 0.5)
c^{amb}	120.11	86.15	118.78	160.31	logNormal(4.77, 0.17)
c^{hosp}	5483.36	3744.44	5394.53	7703.16	logNormal(8.60, 0.18)
c_0^{drug}	110	—	—	—	—
c_1^{drug}	520	—	—	—	—

possible to use different functions to describe the existing knowledge (Robert, 2001).

Conditionally on the relevant elements of $\boldsymbol{\theta}$, the observable health economic response is represented by $Y = (SE_t, A_t, H_t)$. Its joint distribution is specified using the formulation described above and its components can be combined to implement the economic analysis. As discussed in §1.2.1, in general it may or may not be possible to observe directly individual data Y. However, the structure described above can be used in both circumstances and if data are not directly available the predictive distributions can be simulated using the distributional assumptions described above to produce a decision-analytical model.   □

3.3.2   Decision process

Suppose an intervention t is applied and results in the outcome y. In health economic terms, we can quantify this situation by a combination of a measure of clinical effectiveness e (for instance measured in terms of QALYs) of the outcome y, and the costs c associated with the selected intervention t. Thus, as suggested earlier, with each situation (y, t) we associate a pair (e, c). The objective of health economic evaluations is to compare the proposed interventions in terms of their expected performances along these two dimensions of interest, benefit and cost.

For example, we might consider the *increment in mean effectiveness*:

$$\Delta_e := \mathrm{E}[e \mid \theta^1] - \mathrm{E}[e \mid \theta^0]$$

and the *increment in mean cost*:

$$\Delta_c := \mathrm{E}[c \mid \theta^1] - \mathrm{E}[c \mid \theta^0]$$

where the expectations are taken with respect to the distributions of the observable variables (e, c). Note that these are functions of the unknown quantities θ^0, θ^1 and as such, within the Bayesian framework, are random variables. Taking a further expectation with respect to the distribution of $\boldsymbol{\theta}$ produces the quantities defined in (1.2) and (1.3).

The overall utility is $\mathcal{U}^* := \max_t \mathcal{U}^t$, based on choosing the intervention t yielding this maximum value. Equivalently, we choose $t = 1$ if (and, henceforth ignoring ties, only if) EIB > 0, where

$$\mathrm{EIB} := \mathcal{U}^1 - \mathcal{U}^0 \tag{3.3}$$

is the *expected incremental benefit* (of treatment 1 over treatment 0). It is easy to see that

$$\mathcal{U}^* = \max\{\mathrm{EIB}, 0\} + \mathcal{U}^0. \tag{3.4}$$

Note that EIB is a fixed quantity, uncertainty in both domains having been averaged out.

3.3.3 Choosing a utility function: The net benefit

The main difficulty in applying decision theory and (3.2) is that a form of the utility function must be specified. In a health economic problem, we need to combine the two quantities e and c into a single real-valued utility measure, $u(y, t) = f(e, c)$. While there are many possibilities, a common form of utility function is the *(monetary) net benefit* (Stinnett and Mullahy, 1998)

$$u(y, t) = ke - c. \tag{3.5}$$

Here k is a willingness-to-pay parameter (cfr. §1.7) used to put cost and benefits on the same scale and represents the budget that the decision-maker is willing to invest to increase the benefits by one unit.

The main advantage of the net benefit over other possible forms of utility function (and the main reason for its widespread use) is that it has a fixed form, once the variables (e, c) are defined. Moreover, the net benefit is linear in (e, c), which facilitates interpretation and calculations. Nevertheless, the use of the net benefit presupposes that the decision-maker is *risk neutral*, which is by no means always appropriate in health policy problems (Koerkamp et al., 2007). We consider this in more detail in §3.7.1 below.

When the net benefit is used as a utility function, cost-effectiveness analysis focusses on

$$\mathrm{EIB} = \mathrm{E}[k\Delta_e - \Delta_c] = k\mathrm{E}[\Delta_e] - \mathrm{E}[\Delta_c] \tag{3.6}$$

where the expectations are now over the distribution of $\boldsymbol{\theta}$. Equation (3.6) has clear connections with the ICER defined in equation (1.4). In particular, it is easy to show that if EIB > 0 then

$$k > \frac{\mathrm{E}[\Delta_c]}{\mathrm{E}[\Delta_e]} = \mathrm{ICER}$$

and therefore, as suggested in §1.7.1, interventions for which the ICER is less than the willingness-to-pay threshold are considered cost-effective.

Example (continued)

In order to perform the economic analysis, we need to define suitable measures of cost and effectiveness. The total cost associated with each treatment can be computed by multiplying the unit cost of each clinical resource (drugs, ambulatory care and hospital admission) by the number of patients consuming it. Thus

$$c_t := c_t^{\mathrm{drug}}(N - SE_t) + (c_t^{\mathrm{drug}} + c^{\mathrm{amb}})A_t + (c_t^{\mathrm{drug}} + c^{\mathrm{hosp}})H_t.$$

As for the measure of effectiveness, we compute it as the total number of patients who do not experience side effects

$$e_t := (N - SE_t).$$

The model described in §3.3.1 can be run using an MCMC approach to produce a sample from the posterior distribution of (e, c) under the two alternative interventions. Using the results obtained by a large number S of simulations from the model after convergence to the posterior distribution has been assessed, we can compute the expected utility $\mathcal{U}^t$. For example, if we consider the net benefit as utility function, this can be obtained by an MC estimation:

$$\mathcal{U}^t \approx \frac{1}{S}\left[k \sum_{s=1}^{S} e_t^{(s)} - \sum_{s=1}^{S} c_t^{(s)} \right],$$

where $e_t^{(s)}$ and $c_t^{(s)}$ are the s−th simulated value for the measure of effectiveness and cost.

Since it is likely that the decision-maker is not certain about the value of the willingness-to-pay that they will select in a given problem, the analysis is typically performed (and reported) on a grid of reasonable k values. In this case, we select $k \in [0 - 50\,000]$.

The R package BCEA[1] (Baio, 2012) can be used to systematically compute all the relevant syntheses of the economic evaluation process, once the Bayesian model has been run (e.g., but not necessarily, by means of an MCMC approach).

---

[1]Additional information about the package is available at the webpage www.statistica.it/gianluca/BCEA.

We assume here that the simulations from the posterior distributions of interest are available in the R workspace as two matrices e and c, each of dimension $(n_{sim} \times n_{int})$, where n_{sim} is the number of simulations saved and n_{int} is the number of interventions being compared[2] (Chapter 4 discusses how to run a Bayesian model, store and post-process its results using R).

In this case, $n_{int} = 2$ since we are comparing two interventions and we use $n_{sim} = 500$ simulations. The relevant health economic quantities can be produced by running the function bcea, by means of the following commands (cfr. §4.7 for a more detailed description).

```
treats <- c("Old Chemotherapy","New Chemotherapy")
m <- bcea(e=e,c=c,ref=2,interventions=treats,Kmax=50000)
```

The first command defines a vector of labels to be associated with each intervention. Then we create an object m which contains the results of the cost-effectiveness analysis performed by bcea.

This function takes several inputs: the most important ones are the two matrices e and c. Then we need to specify the reference intervention: in this case we set the option ref=2 which tells R that the second column of e and c contains the values simulated for the intervention being compared to the standard treatment. If the option ref is left unspecified, R assumes that the first intervention is to be used as the intervention under analysis.

Next we specify that the interventions have labels defined in the vector treats; if the option interventions was left unspecified, R would construct labels in the form "Intervention 1", ..., "Intervention T" (with T $= n_{int}$).

The last option is related to the willingness-to-pay parameter and specifies the maximum value to be used for the analysis. In this case, we set the option Kmax=50000, which instructs R to select a grid of values between 0 and 50 000. The grid is built by considering a point every Kmax/500 in that interval. If nothing is specified for Kmax, the function bcea automatically considers a value of 50 000.

All the results derived upon varying k in the grid are stored in the object m and the vector of values for k is saved in the element[3] m$k, which in this case contains the 501 values $(0, 500, 1000, \ldots, 50\,000)$.

Using the output produced by bcea and saved in m, we can simply obtain a graph of the cost-effectiveness plane by entering the command ceplane.plot(m,comparison=1,wtp=25000). The input of this function is the object m and there are two possible options: the first one specifies which comparison should be plotted. In this case, there are only two interventions and

---

[2]Notice that, while specifically designed for a Bayesian analysis, BCEA can also be run in a frequentist setting, provided that the two matrices with simulations from the distributions of *e* and *c* are available. In a non-Bayesian setting, these might be obtained, for example, by using re-sampling algorithms such as the bootstrap (although, of course, in that instance they would not represent the posterior distributions).

[3]In R, the elements contained in an object can be accessed using the notation object$element. Thus, typing m$k prints the entire grid of values selected for the willingness-to-pay defined in the object m.

therefore there can only be one comparison. In general, there are $n_{int} - 1$ possible comparisons. The second option specifies the value of the willingness-to-pay to use as reference. In this case, we have chosen the default value of $k = 25\,000$, which is usually recommended by NICE as the reference cost-per-QALY.

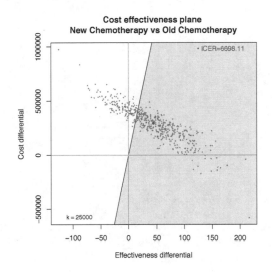

FIGURE 3.1
Cost-effectiveness plane for the chemotherapy example. The dots represent the simulations from the posterior distribution of (Δ_e, Δ_c), while the shaded part of the graph shows the "sustainability area," i.e. the portion of the plane in which the points are below the willingness-to-pay threshold, which is set to 25 000 in this case.

The result is depicted in Figure 3.1, in which the dots are the simulations from the posterior distribution of (Δ_e, Δ_c). The graph also shows the line obtained in correspondence of the set value of k. The shaded area below the line represent the portion of the plane where the simulated values are below that threshold and therefore it can be considered as a "sustainability area."

The red dot represents the ICER (cfr. §1.7). As in this case it lies in the sustainability area, we can conclude that, at the willingness-to-pay threshold selected, the new drug is a cost-effective alternative with respect to the status quo. With respect to Figure 1.6, the current analysis also presents a quantification of the uncertainty underlying the point estimation represented by the ICER, because it is based on the entire distribution of (Δ_e, Δ_c), rather than just on its expectations.

A more comprehensive analysis is provided by Figure 3.2, which is produced by entering the command `eib.plot(m)` in R and depicts the EIB. From the graph, it is possible to identify the *break-even point*, i.e. the value of k

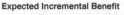

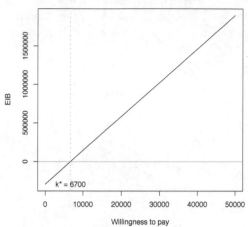

FIGURE 3.2
Analysis of the expected incremental benefit EIB upon varying the willingness-to-pay parameter. For $k < k^* := 6\,700$, EIB < 0 and therefore the status quo is the most cost-effective option. However, if the decision-maker is willing to invest a value exceeding the break-even point of 6 700, then EIB > 0, which implies that the new chemotherapy drug becomes the most cost-effective strategy.

for which the optimal decision is modified. In this case, for $k \leq k^* \approx 6\,700$, EIB < 0 and therefore maintaining the status quo is the optimal decision. Conversely, for all $k > k^*$ the new drug is the most cost-effective strategy. The value of the break-even point corresponds to the ICER and quantifies the point in which the decision-maker is indifferent between the two options. The value of 6 700 is the grid approximation to the ICER.

The R command `summary(m,wtp=25000)` will produce the following summary table.

```
Cost-effectiveness analysis summary

Reference intervention: New Chemotherapy
Comparator intervention: Old Chemotherapy

Optimal decision: choose Old Chemotherapy for k<6700 and
                         New Chemotherapy for k>=6700


Analysis for willingness to pay parameter k = 25000

                  Expected utility
Old Chemotherapy        18608376
```

```
New Chemotherapy          19410840

                                   EIB   CEAC   ICER
New Chemotherapy vs Old Chemotherapy 802465 0.728 6698.1

Optimal intervention (max expected utility) for k=25000: New Chemotherapy

EVPI 237560
```

The summary table provides information about the decision process for the value selected for the input wtp of the willingness-to-pay (some of the quantities presented in the table will be discussed in the next sections). If the decision-maker were willing to set this particular value of k as the budget to allocate for the treatment of the disease under analysis, the EIB for $t = 1$ vs $t = 0$ would be 802 465 for the entire population. Consequently, the new drug would prove to be the most cost-effective intervention and it should be then selected to replace the status quo.   □

3.3.4   Uncertainty in the decision process

The above analysis shows how, in the Bayesian approach, both individual variations and uncertainty in the value of the parameters are averaged out. From the decision-theoretic point of view, identification of the overall expected utility is all that is needed to reach the best decision given the current state of knowledge available to the decision-maker. This point has been argued in the context of health economics by Claxton (1999b) and Claxton et al. (2000).

However, implementing an intervention is typically associated with some risks such as the irreversibility of investments (Claxton, 1999b), and therefore medical decision making can be viewed as a two-stage decision problem (Briggs et al., 2006). If gathering additional data to supplement the background information $\mathcal{D}$ is not an option, the decision-maker must choose now whether to keep the standard programme $t = 0$, or to switch to the new one on the basis of some suitable cost-effectiveness measure of utility (e.g., the net benefit).

However, if deferring the final decision in order first to gather more data is an available option, then the standard intervention $t = 0$ will typically be maintained while additional evidence $\mathcal{E}$ is collected, with the aim of resolving, at least partially, current uncertainty about the parameter $\boldsymbol{\theta}$. Once this evidence is available, the analysis can be updated and the utility for each possible intervention will be based on the new posterior density of the parameters of interest, $p(\theta^t \mid \mathcal{D}, \mathcal{E})$, which will induce a predictive distribution for some other future outcomes z (generally of the same nature as y). The option of postponing the decision on cost-effectiveness is typically associated with additional sampling costs. Figure 3.3 shows a graphical representation of the decision process just described.

For these reasons, it has been advocated in the literature that health economic evaluations should be subjected to some form of Sensitivity Analysis

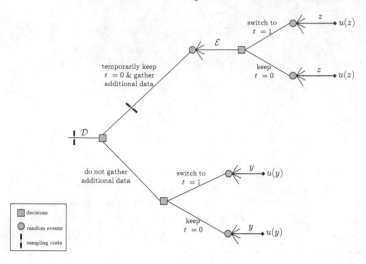

FIGURE 3.3

A graphical representation of the sequential decision problem, in terms of a decision tree.

(SA), in order to quantify and qualify the uncertainty underlying the decision process. Formally, SA is defined in risk assessment as the study of "how uncertainty in some model output can be apportioned, qualitatively or quantitatively, to different sources of uncertainty in the model input" (Saltelli et al., 2004).

Various different forms of SA have been recognised in the health economic literature (Parmigiani, 2002b). *Marginalisation* is implicit in Bayesian decision-theoretic procedures, such as (3.2); the relevant input can be represented by the value of the parameters of the model, $\boldsymbol{\theta}$, whereas the output is the future health economic outcomes on some reference unit. The uncertainty in all the random quantities is accounted for by the computation of the expected utilities used to determine the optimal decision, but is not analysed separately.

The second form of SA is *Scenario Analysis* (sometimes referred to as *Deterministic Sensitivity Analysis*, DSA). In this case, the experimenter selects a list of interesting values for (some of) the parameters of the model and evaluates the expected outcomes under all these different scenarios. This procedure is easy to implement, especially when the number of parameters involved is relatively small. However, it fails to consider the possible correlation or the underlying uncertainty about the parameters of interest, only focusing on a set of arbitrarily chosen values, regardless of the likelihood of each of them occurring in reality.

3.4 Probabilistic sensitivity analysis to parameter uncertainty

These limitations can be overcome by *Probabilistic Sensitivity Analysis* (PSA), a procedure in which all input parameters are considered as random quantities and are therefore associated with a probability distribution that describes the state of science (i.e. the background knowledge of the decision-maker). This method is in line with the Bayesian analysis, but, instead of being marginalised out, as required by the decision-theoretic analysis, the uncertainty in the parameters is explicitly analysed by means of suitable indicators.

To understand the rationale behind PSA, consider a situation in which the information provided by the evidence $\mathcal{D}$ is so accurate that $p(\boldsymbol{\theta} \mid \mathcal{D})$ is close to a one-point distribution at the true value: in this case, we shall have effectively learned $\boldsymbol{\theta}$. In other words, the uncertainty on the knowledge domain will be totally resolved.

If we then adopt intervention t, the "known-distribution" expected utility will be

$$
\begin{aligned}
U(\theta^t) \quad &:= \quad \mathrm{E}[u(Y,t) \mid \mathcal{D}] \\
&= \quad \int u(y,t)\, p(y \mid \theta^t)\, dy.
\end{aligned}
\tag{3.7}
$$

Consequently, the overall utility is $U^*(\boldsymbol{\theta}) := \max_t U(\theta^t)$ and we would choose treatment $t = 1$ if $U(\theta^1) > U(\theta^0)$, or equivalently if $\mathrm{IB}(\boldsymbol{\theta}) > 0$, where

$$
\mathrm{IB}(\boldsymbol{\theta}) := U(\theta^1) - U(\theta^0)
\tag{3.8}
$$

is the *incremental benefit* under parameter-pair $\boldsymbol{\theta}$. Note that, similarly to equation (3.4), we have

$$
U^*(\boldsymbol{\theta}) = \max\{\mathrm{IB}(\boldsymbol{\theta}), 0\} + U(\theta^0).
\tag{3.9}
$$

Obviously, in general we shall not be able to learn the value of $\boldsymbol{\theta}$ with certainty. For this reason, $\mathrm{IB}(\boldsymbol{\theta})$ and $U(\theta^t)$ remain random quantities, whose current probability distributions are induced by $p(\boldsymbol{\theta} \mid \mathcal{D})$.

The idea behind PSA is to compare the *actual* decision process, based on the analysis of EIB and (3.3), to the *ideal* one, characterised by the (currently unknown) quantities computed in equations (3.7) and (3.8). This is done with a view to assessing whether the information provided by the current evidence $\mathcal{D}$ is sufficient to take a decision on the optimal treatment, or it would be more effective to defer the final decision until after additional evidence $\mathcal{E}$ is collected.

Although analytical methods have also been described (Oakley and O'Hagan, 2004; Oakley, 2009), PSA is typically conducted using a simulation approach (Doubilet et al., 1985). For each of a sequence of iterations

$s = 1, \ldots, S$, a value $\boldsymbol{\theta}_{(s)}$ is simulated from the distribution $p(\boldsymbol{\theta} \mid \mathcal{D})$. The decision analysis is then conducted using that specific value *as if* this were the realised one. By means of this procedure, it is possible to produce a sample from the distribution of $U(\theta^t)$, IB$(\boldsymbol{\theta})$ or any other related random quantity; the resulting variability in the expected utilities and the influence of each component of $\boldsymbol{\theta}$ can then be suitably summarised.

Example (continued)

Table 3.2 shows the results of the simulation exercise described in §3.3.3. For each of the 500 iterations, we simulated values for all the parameters (shown in the upper half of Table 3.2) from the distributions defined or induced by Table 3.1.

Considering the net benefit as a utility function, we can rewrite (3.7) and (3.8) respectively as

$$U(\theta^t) = k\mathrm{E}[e \mid \theta^t] - \mathrm{E}[c \mid \theta^t] \tag{3.10}$$

and

$$\mathrm{IB}(\boldsymbol{\theta}) = k\Delta_e - \Delta_c. \tag{3.11}$$

and use the simulated values for the parameters to calculate the expected utility of option t that would be obtained if the uncertainty on the parameters were resolved to the specific values simulated, which are shown in the lower half of Table 3.2, which can be obtained using the BCEA function sim.table(m,wtp=25000).

While this process can be repeated for each value of k, in Table 3.2 we show again the computations for the reference value of $k = 25\,000$. The last row of the table reports the average values computed over all the simulations of the model, while the last two columns are described in details in §3.5.2.

For all the values of k in m$k, the elements m$U, m$Ustar and m$ib contain respectively: the known-distribution utilities for all the interventions being compared, $U(\theta^t)$; the known-distribution maximum utility, $U^*(\boldsymbol{\theta})$; and the values of the incremental benefit IB$(\boldsymbol{\theta})$.   □

3.5   Reporting the results of probabilistic sensitivity analysis

Much of the recent theoretical work in health economics has been devoted specifically to the issue of reporting the results of PSA using suitable summary measures (Briggs et al., 2002; Parmigiani, 2002a; O'Hagan et al., 2004; Claxton et al., 2005; Griffin et al., 2006; O'Hagan et al., 2006). As suggested earlier, while the process of marginalisation performed computing the expected

TABLE 3.2

PSA in practice. For each iteration, we first simulate a value for the parameters $\boldsymbol{\theta}$ from the distributions described in Table 3.1. These are shown in the upper part of this table. Then (lower part of this table), for each intervention and for each iteration s of the model the induced expected utilities are calculated, according to (3.10) and (3.11), and using a fixed value of $k = 25\,000$; for each iteration, the maximum expected utility (*i.e.* of the optimal intervention) is typeset in italics. The last two columns of the lower part of this table are computed according to (3.12) and (3.14). For each column, the average is computed over the rows (model simulations).

s	π_0	π_1	ρ	γ	c^{amb}	c^{hosp}	SE_0	SE_1	A_0	A_1	H_0	H_1
1	0.28	0.29	1.04	0.65	103.6	6012.4	274	267	134	132	140	135
2	0.22	0.05	0.21	0.63	142.4	4076.9	221	144	126	78	95	66
3	0.22	0.15	0.68	0.63	119.8	5452.9	225	262	90	98	135	164
4	0.16	0.21	1.32	0.64	89.6	7863.8	255	105	171	71	84	34
5	0.25	0.21	0.85	0.65	97.5	4483.4	188	151	123	100	65	51
6	0.30	0.13	0.44	0.60	118.9	5039.4	245	218	117	100	128	118
...						...						...
500	0.23	0.19	0.80	0.59	130.1	5678.5	205	178	91	79	114	99

s	$U(\theta^0)$	$U(\theta^1)$	$U^*(\boldsymbol{\theta})$	$\mathrm{IB}(\boldsymbol{\theta})$	$\mathrm{OL}(\boldsymbol{\theta})$	$\mathrm{VI}(\boldsymbol{\theta})$
1	*17305384*	17096285	17305384	−209099	209099	−17972570
2	18873525	*20539653*	20539653	1666127	—	39592192
3	*18440423*	16929833	18440423	−1510590	1510590	10821981
4	17969992	*21634230*	21634230	3664238	—	13138737
5	19732495	*20345594*	20345594	613099	—	−2626805
6	18241461	*18548107*	18548107	306646	—	16302580
...			...			...
500	18745045	*19144252*	19144252	399206	—	−266588
Average	$\mathcal{U}^0 =$	$\mathcal{U}^1 =$	$\mathcal{V}^* =$	$\mathrm{EIB} =$	$\mathrm{EVPI} =$	$\mathrm{EVPI} =$
	185204459	*19410840*	19648400	802464.54	237559.92	237559.92

utilities $\mathcal{U}^t$ provides the "best" decision given the current data, the essence of PSA is to use the induced distributions for the health economic indicators to qualify the extent to which uncertainty impacts on the decision process. We next review the main indicators used to this end, clarifying the basic differences in their nature.

3.5.1 Cost-effectiveness acceptability curves

In health economic evaluations it is common to summarise the results of PSA by means of the *cost-effectiveness acceptability curve* (CEAC, Van Hout et al.,

1994), defined as:

$$\text{CEAC} = \text{Pr}(\text{IB}(\boldsymbol{\theta}) > 0).$$

If the net benefit is used as a utility function, this can be re-expressed as $\text{CEAC} = \text{Pr}(k\Delta_e - \Delta_c > 0)$, which depends on the willingness-to-pay parameter k. When EIB > 0, i.e. the optimal decision is treatment 1, this is the probability that learning the value of $\boldsymbol{\theta}$ (i.e. resolving the uncertainty on the parameters) would not change that decision.

By their very nature, CEACs provide a simple synthesis of the uncertainty about the cost-effectiveness of a given intervention (Fenwick et al., 2001) and have been widely used in the health economics literature (Briggs, 2000; O'Hagan et al., 2000; O'Brien and Briggs, 2002; Parmigiani, 2002b; Spiegelhalter and Best, 2003).

The main advantage of CEACs is that they allow a simple summarisation of the probability of cost-effectiveness upon varying the willingness-to-pay parameter, effectively performing a DSA on k. This circumstance proves to be particularly useful in presenting the results of economic analysis, as decision-makers are often not ready to commit to a single value of k (i.e. a single utility function) prior to the analysis being performed.

In particular, if the net benefit is used as utility function, the CEAC represents the probability that the intervention $t = 1$ is cheaper if $k \to 0$; conversely, for $k \to \infty$, i.e. Δ_c is effectively irrelevant in the computation of probabilities for IB$(\boldsymbol{\theta})$, the CEAC represents the probability that $t = 1$ is more effective than $t = 0$.

Example (continued)

For the example of §3.3.1, Figure 3.4 shows the CEAC, again upon varying the value of the parameter k in the range $[0; 50,000]$. This graph can be obtained by simply running the R function `ceac.plot(m)`, which is part of BCEA.

For relatively small values of k the probability of cost-effectiveness is low, indicating higher uncertainty in the actual cost-effectiveness of the new drug (or, equivalently, low uncertainty in the cost-effectiveness of the comparator). This makes sense, as the preferred option in this range of k is the status quo. For $k \approx 6\,700$ the CEAC reaches a value of 0.5 (when the uncertainty as to which is the most cost-effective intervention is maximum).

Figure 3.4 seems to suggest that for large values of k, the probability that choosing it is the "correct" decision is increasingly higher and is 0.73 for $k = 25\,000$. This figure can be deduced from (the complete version of) Table 3.2 as the proportion of simulations for which IB$(\boldsymbol{\theta}) > 0$ — cfr. equation (3.8). The values of the CEAC are stored in R in the element `m$ceac`. □

Despite their wide use, some critical limitations have been pointed out (Fenwick et al., 2004), the main one being that CEACs do not contain a decision rule. For instance, they can only address the problem of *how likely*

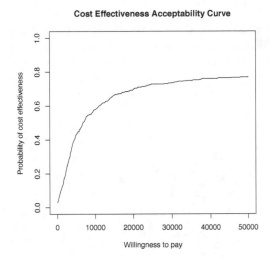

Cost Effectiveness Acceptability Curve

FIGURE 3.4

PSA by means of the analysis of the CEAC. For each value of the willingness-to-pay parameter k, the CEAC is computed as the proportion of simulations for which $IB(\boldsymbol{\theta}) > 0$. Higher values for the CEAC indicate that, for a given budget that the decision-maker is willing to invest, the probability that vaccination is in fact more cost-effective than the status quo is large.

it is that resolving parameters' uncertainty will change the optimal decision (Felli and Hazen, 1999). However, no explicit reference is made to the *possible change in the payoffs*.

More recently, it has been suggested that very different distributions for the IB can produce the same value of the CEAC, which makes it difficult to interpret and might lead to incorrect conclusions for policy makers (Koerkamp et al., 2007).

Consider for example two very simple economic models: model (a) is characterised by the following assumptions:

- $E(\Delta_c) = £1\,100$; $sd(\Delta_c) = £1\,100$;

- $E(\Delta_e) = 0.05$ QALYs; $sd(\Delta_e) = 0.05$ QALYs;

- $Corr(\Delta_c, \Delta_e) = 0$.

Model (b), on the other hand, is defined so that:

- $E(\Delta_c) = £11\,000$; $sd(\Delta_c) = £11\,000$

- $E(\Delta_e) = 0.5$ QALYs; $sd(\Delta_e) = 0.5$ QALYs;

• $\mathrm{Corr}(\Delta_c, \Delta_e) = 0$.

Using for instance a simulative procedure, it is possible to obtain a sample of values from the distributions of the differentials of costs and effectiveness by means of which it is possible to analyse the cost-effectiveness plane for both models. Figure 3.5 shows the result of 1000 simulations from the two models for a fixed value of $k = £25\,000$.

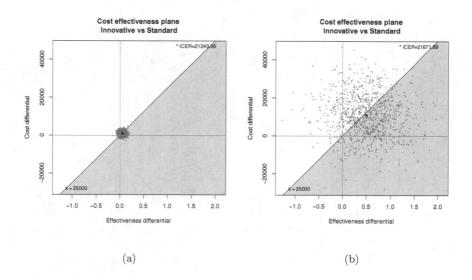

(a)   (b)

FIGURE 3.5
PSA by means of CEAC in two separate models: the value of the CEAC is the same, despite the fact that the two models are substantially different in terms of the associated variability.

As is possible to see, the two distributions are substantially different: model (a) shows absolute values that are much lower than those of model (b); more importantly, the variability associated with the estimations of (Δ_e, Δ_c) is quite different. However, the proportion of points below the line identifying the value of k (i.e. the CEAC) is the same in both cases (and equals 0.53 in this example).

Finally, CEACs are concerned only with currently available information, but do not consider explicitly the possibility of gathering additional evidence. Consequently, by means of CEACs only a partial evaluation of the overall decision process is provided. For this reason, if sensitivity analysis is performed in the context described above (i.e., with the possibility of deferring the decision), the use of CEACs alone is not ideal.

3.5.2 The value of information

A purely decision-theoretic approach to PSA, avoiding the shortcomings of CEACs, is based on the *value of information* analysis (Howard, 1966), an increasingly popular method in health economic evaluations (Felli and Hazen, 1998, 1999; Claxton, 1999a; Claxton et al., 2001; Ades et al., 2004; Brennan and Kharroubi, 2005; Briggs et al., 2006; Fenwick et al., 2006). In this approach, we compare the overall value of the decision process in the ideal scenario, represented by $U^*(\boldsymbol{\theta})$, to that obtained in the actual evaluation, $\mathcal{U}^*$.

The value of obtaining information on $\boldsymbol{\theta}$ is defined as

$$\mathrm{VI}(\boldsymbol{\theta}) := U^*(\boldsymbol{\theta}) - \mathcal{U}^*, \tag{3.12}$$

which for each value of $\boldsymbol{\theta}$ quantifies the difference in the utilities produced by the information on the parameters.

Again, since in general the value of $U^*(\boldsymbol{\theta})$ cannot be determined with certainty, we synthesise its distribution considering the *expected value of "perfect" information*

$$
\begin{aligned}
\mathrm{EVPI} \quad &:= \quad \mathrm{E}\left[\mathrm{VI}(\boldsymbol{\theta})\right] \\
&= \quad \int \mathrm{VI}(\boldsymbol{\theta})\, p(\boldsymbol{\theta} \mid \mathcal{D})\, d\boldsymbol{\theta} \\
&= \quad \mathcal{V}^* - \mathcal{U}^*, \tag{3.13}
\end{aligned}
$$

where

$$\mathcal{V}^* := \mathrm{E}\left[U^*(\boldsymbol{\theta})\right] = \int U^*(\boldsymbol{\theta})\, p(\boldsymbol{\theta} \mid \mathcal{D})\, d\boldsymbol{\theta}$$

is the expectation of the overall known-distribution utility $U^*(\boldsymbol{\theta})$. Notice that the additional information that may become available need not be "perfect". In other words, we might not be able to learn the value of a parameter perfectly, although new data will generally make our estimation more precise, therefore leading to a less variable posterior distribution. Extensions of this argument are sometimes developed in terms of expected value of *sample* information, EVSI (Ades et al., 2004).

If $\tau = \arg\max_t \mathcal{U}^t$ is the intervention associated with the overall maximum expected utility, for each value of $\boldsymbol{\theta}$ we can consider

$$\mathrm{OL}(\boldsymbol{\theta}) := U^*(\boldsymbol{\theta}) - U(\theta^\tau), \tag{3.14}$$

the *opportunity loss* derived by choosing the alternative associated with the highest overall expected utility, instead of the one associated with the highest known-distribution utility. As is easy to see, the average value of $\mathrm{OL}(\boldsymbol{\theta})$ coincides with the value of EVPI:

$$
\begin{aligned}
\mathrm{E}[\mathrm{OL}(\boldsymbol{\theta})] \quad &= \quad \int \left[U^*(\boldsymbol{\theta}) - U(\theta^\tau)\right] p(\boldsymbol{\theta} \mid \mathcal{D})\, d\boldsymbol{\theta} \\
&= \quad \int U^*(\boldsymbol{\theta})\, p(\boldsymbol{\theta} \mid \mathcal{D})\, d\boldsymbol{\theta} - \int U(\theta^\tau)\, p(\theta^\tau \mid \mathcal{D})\, d\theta^\tau \\
&= \quad \mathcal{V}^* - \mathcal{U}^* = \mathrm{EVPI}.
\end{aligned}
$$

While the value of information $\text{VI}(\boldsymbol{\theta})$ can take on negative values, the opportunity loss $\text{OL}(\boldsymbol{\theta})$ is necessarily non-negative. Consequently, by a simple application of Jensen's inequality, it can be proved that the EVPI is a non-negative quantity as well.

The EVPI places an upper limit to the amount that the decision-maker would be willing to pay to obtain any information, perfect or imperfect, about $\boldsymbol{\theta}$. By construction, it measures the *weighted average opportunity loss* induced by the decision based on the EIB, the weight being the probability of incurring that loss. Therefore, this measure gives us an appropriately integrated indication of: (a) *how much* we are likely to lose if we take the "wrong" decision, and (b) *how likely* it is that we take it, as is easily appreciated using (3.4) and (3.9) to re-express (3.13) as

$$
\begin{aligned}
\text{EVPI} \;&=\; \text{E}\left[U^*(\boldsymbol{\theta}) - \mathcal{U}^*\right] \\
&=\; \text{E}\left[\max\{\text{IB}(\boldsymbol{\theta}), 0\}\right] - \max\{\text{EIB}, 0\} \\
&=\; \text{E}\left[\text{IB}(\boldsymbol{\theta}) \mid \text{IB}(\boldsymbol{\theta}) > 0\right] \times \Pr(\text{IB}(\boldsymbol{\theta}) > 0) - \max\{\text{EIB}, 0\} \\
&=\; \text{E}\left[\text{IB}(\boldsymbol{\theta}) \mid \text{IB}(\boldsymbol{\theta}) > 0\right] \times \text{CEAC} - \max\{\text{EIB}, 0\}
\end{aligned}
$$

(the expectations are all taken with respect to the joint distribution of $\boldsymbol{\theta}$).

If $\text{EIB} > 0$ then selecting the treatment $t = 0$ just because (from the analysis of CEAC) there is a large variability in $\text{IB}(\boldsymbol{\theta})$ may impose unnecessary losses on society, as patients may miss out on a potentially cost-effective treatment (Claxton, 1999b). In contrast, the EVPI analysis provides the decision-maker with a rational procedure overcoming this problem. If the large variability in $\text{IB}(\boldsymbol{\theta})$ is associated with low cost for additional research, then the decision-maker can postpone the decision, or perhaps select the treatment $t = 1$ only for a subset of the population.

For example, Figure 3.6 shows the analysis of the EIB and EVPI for the two models compared in Figure 3.5. Because the ratios $\text{E}(\Delta_c)/\text{E}(\Delta_e)$ are the same in the two models, the break even points coincide (minor differences are due to the simulation variability). However, the utilities are substantially different, since in model (b) the costs and effects are ten times higher than in model (a). Unlike the CEAC, the EVPI is sensitive to this aspect: the payoffs in model (b) are much larger and therefore the impact of uncertainty on the decision process is much higher. This is reflected in values of the EVPI that are ten times higher than those of model (a).

The value of information analysis is sometimes considered as a separate methodology, which can be performed independently on PSA. However, in our view, for the reasons explained above, it is a fundamental part of the sensitivity analysis process and is in line with the objective of identifying and quantifying the impact of parameters' uncertainty on the decision process. Therefore we view it as the proper method to perform PSA.

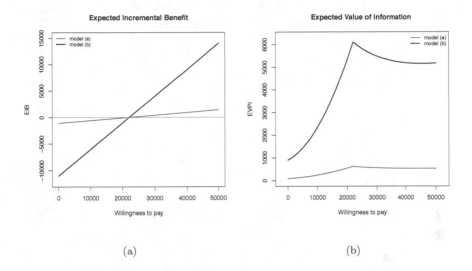

(a) (b)

FIGURE 3.6

PSA by means of EVPI in two separate models: unlike the CEAC, the EVPI is sensitive to the difference in the payoffs associated with the underlying model (cfr. Figure 3.5). Because in model (b) costs and effects are much larger than in model (a), uncertainty has a higher impact on the former.

Example (continued)

Figure 3.7 is produced by the command `evi.plot(m)` and shows the analysis of the population (i.e. for the whole N patients considered) expected value of information as a function of the willingness-to-pay parameter k for the running example. The EVPI changes its shape around the break-even point $k \approx 6\,700$, since the optimal decision is reversed beyond that threshold.

As k increases from 0, the value of reducing uncertainty becomes increasingly larger. Just after the break-even point, it remains almost constant for a few values of k, but then it increases steadily. Even for values of k where there is higher uncertainty in the optimal decision, the absolute magnitude of the patient-specific EVPI (which can be easily computed by dividing the population EVPI by the total number of patients N) is relatively small (compared to the values of the payoffs), in this case. At the maximum level of uncertainty (i.e. when the decision-maker is willing to allocate a budget of £50 000), the expected value of information is about £350 per patient.

For industry-sponsored studies, the overall per-patient cost of a cancer clinical trial has been estimated to vary between $60 000 and $85 000 for Phase III studies (Institute of Medicine, 2008). Thus, as compared to these cost of research (which might be performed to reduce the uncertainty in the parame-

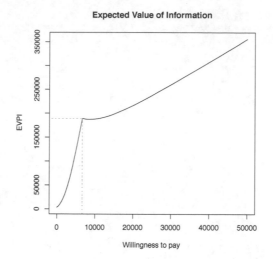

FIGURE 3.7
PSA by means of the analysis of the expected value of information. For each value of the willingness-to-pay parameter k, the EVPI represents the average opportunity loss deriving by using the current most cost-effective intervention, instead of further investigating to reduce the uncertainty in the parameters. Higher values for the EVPI indicate that, for a given budget that the decision-maker is willing to invest, the value of additional research is large.

ters), this implies that uncertainty in the parameters does not have a dramatic impact. Moreover, since the EVPI is less than the expected cost of research, additional evidence would not be beneficial and a decision can be taken based on the currently available information.

Just as for the other main outputs of the economic analysis, for all k, the function bcea stores the value of information $\mathrm{VI}(\boldsymbol{\theta})$, the opportunity loss $\mathrm{OL}(\boldsymbol{\theta})$ and the EVPI in the elements mvi, mol and m$evi, respectively. □

3.5.3   The value of partial information

Often, the analysis of the value of information can be refined by considering as specifically relevant only some of the elements of the parameter vector. In other words, the model might include a vector of parameters $\boldsymbol{\theta} = (\boldsymbol{\phi}, \boldsymbol{\psi})$ — each of these elements may itself be a vector, as a function of the number of treatments to be considered. Sometimes, one of the two elements is considered as a nuisance parameter (cfr. §2.4.4) in the analysis of the value of information.

Suppose that we are interested in the component $\boldsymbol{\phi}$. If we were able to resolve uncertainty on this element, the decision process would be exclusively based on marginalisation of the uncertainty about the remaining random quantities ψ. Thus, the optimal option would be the one associated with the maximum expected utility

$$
\begin{aligned}
U^*(\phi) &= \max_t \mathrm{E}\left[u(Y,t,\psi^t) \mid \mathcal{D},\phi^t\right] \\
&= \max_t \int_{\mathcal{Y}} \int_{\Psi^t} u(y,t,\psi^t)\, p(y,\psi^t \mid \phi^t)\, \mathrm{d}y \mathrm{d}\psi^t \\
&= \max_t \int_{\mathcal{Y}} \int_{\Psi^t} u(y,t,\psi^t)\, p(y \mid \psi^t,\phi^t)\, p(\psi^t \mid \phi^t)\, \mathrm{d}y \mathrm{d}\psi^t \\
&= \max_t \int_{\mathcal{Y}} \int_{\Psi^t} u(y,t,\psi^t)\, p(y \mid \boldsymbol{\theta}^t)\, p(\psi^t \mid \phi^t)\, \mathrm{d}y \mathrm{d}\psi^t .
\end{aligned}
$$

Now, in line with (3.13), it is possible to compute the *expected value of (perfect) partial information* as:

$$
\begin{aligned}
\text{EVPPI} &:= \int_{\Phi} U^*(\phi)\, p(\phi \mid \mathcal{D})\, \mathrm{d}\phi - \mathcal{U}^* \qquad\qquad (3.15) \\
&= \mathcal{V}^*(\phi) - \mathcal{U}^* .
\end{aligned}
$$

Theoretically, computing the EVPPI does not present any further difficulty with respect to the EVPI. However, the computation of (3.15) is generally much more complex because it involves two different levels of marginalisation of the parameters. In fact, it is necessary to compute first the expected value with respect to the conditional distribution $p(\psi \mid \phi)$, which is needed to compute $U^*(\phi)$, and then with respect to the marginal distribution $p(\phi)$, which is used to determine (3.15) — see Brennan et al. (2007) and Coyle and Oakley (2008) for more detailed reviews of the technical aspects related to the calculation of the EVPPI.

A relatively simple (albeit potentially still very intensive from a computational perspective) way of computing the EVPPI is through a simulation approach based on MCMC. This involves a two stages approach: at the first stage, a vector of n_{out} simulations for the parameter of interest ϕ is obtained from the joint posterior distribution $p(\phi,\psi \mid \mathcal{D})$. Then, for each simulated value of ϕ, the model is run again for a large number n_{inn} of simulations. In every run of this second stage, the value of ϕ is fixed to the simulated one, effectively making it a deterministic node. All the other parameters are then estimated from their conditional distribution given $\phi = \phi^{(s)}$, where $\phi^{(s)}$ is the s–th simulated value of the main parameter.

Effectively, this procedure amounts to considering an "outer" cycle (where the value of ϕ is repeatedly simulated) and an "inner" loop (where, conditionally on that value, all the other parameters are simulated). Consequently, in non trivial models this procedure can require a long time to execute.

Example (continued)

Suppose that the main parameter of interest is the decrease in the chance of experiencing side effects with the new drug. Then, in the notation used above, $\phi = \rho$ and $\psi = (\pi_0, \pi_1, \gamma, c^{\text{amb}}, c^{\text{hosp}})$.

We set $n_{\text{out}} = n_{\text{inn}} = 500$. First we run the original model, including the parameter ρ with distributions as in Table 3.1. This produces a vector of simulations from the marginal distribution of ρ, accounting for the uncertainty in the remaining parameters.

Then, for each simulation $s = 1, \ldots, n_{\text{out}}$, we rerun the model producing n_{inn} iterations, this time setting $\pi_1 = \pi_0 \rho^{(s)}$. We then obtain a vector of simulations for ψ, given the fixed value of ϕ. This has an obvious impact especially on π_1, which depends directly on ρ.

For each simulated value of ϕ, we can use the n_{inn} simulations to run the economic analysis. In other words, for each s we first run the MCMC procedure on the model with fixed value of ρ. Then we compute the measures of cost and effectiveness as in §3.3.3 using the n_{inn} simulated values for all the other parameters. Next, we run the function bcea which for each of the n_{inn} iterations computes the known-distribution expected utilities, with which it is easy to compute $U^*(\phi^{(s)})$ by selecting the maximum value. In other words, we end up with a vector of n_{inn} values from the distribution of $U^*(\phi^{(s)})$. By taking the mean of these we obtain $\mathcal{V}^*(\phi)$ and by subtracting the overall maximum expected utility $\mathcal{U}^*$, we can easily compute the EVPPI.

Figure 3.8 shows the EVPPI for ρ together with the overall EVPI. The impact of uncertainty on the parameter ρ is quite substantial and for some values of k the EVPPI is nearly identical with the overall EVPI. This is reasonable as the actual effectiveness of the new treatment obviously depends on the reduction in the occurrence of side effects. Moreover, since the new drug is quite more expensive than the standard, if there is substantial uncertainty on its clinical benefits, the cost-effectiveness profile will be much affected.

A more detailed account of the programming steps required to compute the EVPPI is given in §4.7.1.   □

3.6   Probabilistic sensitivity analysis to structural uncertainty

Recently some research has been devoted to PSA to *structural* uncertainty (Jackson et al., 2009, 2010, 2011; Strong et al., 2011). By this terminology we indicate the situation where a class of different statistical models fitted to the available data is considered to represent the current health economic problem. Thus, uncertainty is present not only on the value of the relevant parameters,

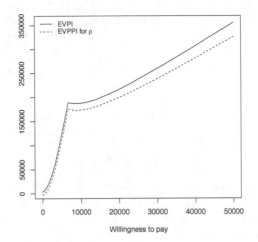

FIGURE 3.8
Analysis of the expected value of partial information: the impact of the parameter ρ on decision uncertainty is quite relevant, as the EVPPI is smaller than the overall EVPI.

but also on which of these models might be the one that best describes the real problem.

The conventional Bayesian way to deal with this issue is by means of *model averaging* (Draper, 1995). This entails defining a finite and exhaustive set of plausible models $\mathcal{M} = (\mathcal{M}_1, \ldots, \mathcal{M}_H)$. In line with the Bayesian framework, for each $h = 1, \ldots, H$ the model is characterised by some parameters $\boldsymbol{\theta}$ that are associated with a suitable prior probability distribution $p(\boldsymbol{\theta} \mid \mathcal{M}_h)$.

However, in addition to the standard setting, a prior probability $p(\mathcal{M}_h)$ that model h is the "true" one is also defined. On the basis of the observed data, the prior over the models is updated to produce a posterior probability

$$p(\mathcal{M}_h \mid y) \propto p(\mathcal{M}_h) \int p(y \mid \boldsymbol{\theta}, \mathcal{M}_h) p(\boldsymbol{\theta} \mid \mathcal{M}_h) \mathrm{d}\boldsymbol{\theta}.$$

The posterior probabilities can be used to compute the average of any function of the parameters (e.g. the utility function defined by the net benefit) over the possible models. Examples of applications of this methodology in the health economic literature include Negrín and Vàzquez-Polo (2008) and Conigliani and Tancredi (2009).

An alternative approach compares different models on the basis of their out-of-sample predictive ability, i.e. on how well the predictive distribution for a given model would fit a replicated dataset based on the observed data

(Jackson et al., 2010). The rationale behind this is that in many applied problems, including health economic evaluations, the possible models that we consider are only a (sometimes quite) rough approximation to the complex phenomenon under study. Thus, there is no guarantee that one of the models in the set $\mathcal{M}$ should be the "true" one.

In line with a decision-theoretic approach, a utility function can be defined for each model to measure the goodness of fit of several alternative specifications. A common measure for Bayesian model comparison is the Deviance Information Criterion (DIC, Spiegelhalter et al., 2002). The DIC is based on the *model deviance*, a likelihood-based measure of model fit defined for a given model as

$$D(\theta) = -2\log p(y \mid \theta),$$

assuming that θ represents the parameters of interest.

Typically, models characterised by a large number of parameters are subjected to "over-fitting", i.e. they tend to fit the observations at hand very well, but generally perform much worse for other similar data. Consequently, they are associated with artificially small values of $D(\theta)$ and thus it is sensible to penalise complexity, if the objective of the analysis is to produce a comparison of the competing models.

A suitable measure of model complexity can be quantified by the function

$$\begin{aligned} p_D &= \mathrm{E}_{\theta|y}[D(\theta)] + D(\mathrm{E}_{\theta|y}[\theta]) \\ &= \bar{D} - D(\bar{\theta}), \end{aligned}$$

representing the "effective number of parameters in the model." In fact, p_D combines the complexity of the structure assumed for the sampling distribution, as well as the strength of the priors. Thus, models associated with strong prior distributions will tend to have smaller values for this statistic. An alternative estimation has been proposed by Gelman et al. (2004) as

$$p_D = \frac{\mathrm{Var}\,[D(\theta)]}{2},$$

which has the advantage of being invariant to parameterisation, robust and trivial to calculate, especially when using MCMC procedures (cfr. Chapter 4).

The DIC is then defined as:

$$\mathrm{DIC} = D(\bar{\theta}) + 2p_D = \bar{D} + p_D. \tag{3.16}$$

Smaller values of the DIC indicate better fit. However, it should be noticed that only differences in the DIC are important, while its absolute size is irrelevant. This is due to the fact that the definition of the model deviance involves a scaling constant (depending only on the data), which is an arbitrary quantity.

Consequently, rather than a method for the formal identification of the "true" model, the DIC is a tool that can be used to compare a collection of alternative model specifications, neither of which may be the correct one.

Moreover, it should be noticed that the DIC has a formal justification for models where the posterior distribution of the parameters of interest is (approximately) Normal. When the sample size is large enough, asymptotic arguments can be brought forward, but for models informed by limited evidence this might be a crucial limitation.

Nevertheless, the DIC is a simple tool, which can be easily obtained as a by-product of MCMC procedures and can be used to produce model-averaged results in a straightforward manner.

If we consider the set of models $\mathcal{M} = (\mathcal{M}_1, \ldots, \mathcal{M}_H)$, we can compute the value DIC_h for each of them and derive the respective weights (i.e. the model posterior probabilities) by simply re-proportioning them, for instance as

$$w_h = \frac{\exp(-0.5\Delta\text{DIC}_h)}{\sum\limits_{h=1}^{H} \exp(-0.5\Delta\text{DIC}_h)}, \tag{3.17}$$

where $\Delta\text{DIC}_h = \min\limits_h (\text{DIC}_h) - \text{DIC}_h$. Notice that equation (3.17) represents only *a* possibility to derive the weights to be attached to each model under consideration. To our knowledge, no extensive research has been done into the properties of this strategy and thus it should not be used uncritically.

The weights w_h can be used to build an average model which accounts for all the possible *posited* data generating processes still considering the possibility that none of these actually is the real one. For example, the outputs of the H models can be combined into a single set of variables obtained as weighted averages of the individual model's results.

Example (continued)

Consider the cost-effectiveness model for the chemotherapy drug presented in §3.3.1, which we indicate with $\mathcal{M}_1$. In addition to that, we now explicitly account for the situation where in fact the new drug does not produce a reduction in the occurrence of the side effects. In fact we assume that the "true" effectiveness of the two alternatives is the same, which is translated in a new model, say $\mathcal{M}_2$, in which $\rho = 1$, with no uncertainty, all other model characteristics being equal.

We then replicate the health economic analysis based on the new model and some synthetical results are presented in Figure 3.9.

As is possible to see, all the simulated values for (Δ_c, Δ_e) lie in the north-eastern or north-western quadrants of the cost-effectiveness plane. This means that under $\mathcal{M}_2$ the probability that the new treatment produces a reduction in costs is effectively 0. This is reasonable, since the innovative drug has a much higher acquisition cost and we are imposing no significant difference in the measure of effectiveness.

Consequently, under $\mathcal{M}_2$ the status quo is the most cost-effective alternative for all values of the willingness-to-pay that we consider, as is confirmed

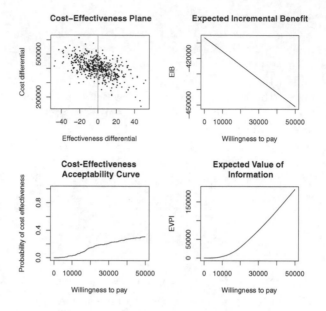

FIGURE 3.9
Synthesis of the health economic analysis for $\mathcal{M}_2$. The four panels present the cost-effectiveness plane, and the analysis of the EIB, CEAC and EVPI upon varying the value of the willingness-to-pay threshold in the interval $[0; 50\,000]$.

by the analysis of the EIB, which is negative throughout the grid of k-values. This of course has a clear impact on the CEAC, which has very low values. Uncertainty on the optimality of $t = 0$ is relatively limited, since the EVPI reaches a maximum value of about $200\,000$ (i.e. only £200 per patient).

The DIC is 42.35784 and 43.25439 respectively for $\mathcal{M}_1$ and $\mathcal{M}_2$. Thus, using (3.17) the model weights can be computed as $w_1 = 0.61023$ and $w_2 = 0.38977$.

Finally, we can compute an "average" model by mixing the simulations coming from $\mathcal{M}_1$ and $\mathcal{M}_2$ with weights w_1 and w_2; for example, for each MCMC simulation s, we can compute the number of individuals presenting side effects as

$$SE_{\text{avg}}^{(s)} = w_1 SE_1^{(s)} + w_2 SE_2^{(s)},$$

where $SE_h^{(s)}$ is the corresponding value simulated at iteration s in model $\mathcal{M}_h$ ($h = 1, 2$). Using similar reasoning, it is possible to build suitable variables of cost and effectiveness for the "average" model, which can be used to rerun the health economic analysis to produce the results depicted in Figure 3.10.

As is obvious, the model average considers the results from both $\mathcal{M}_1$ and $\mathcal{M}_2$: thus, the break-even point is slightly higher than in the original analysis,

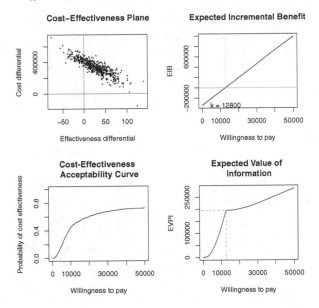

FIGURE 3.10
Synthesis of the health economic analysis for the model average. The results are obtained by averaging the two models $\mathcal{M}_1$ and $\mathcal{M}_2$. The break-even point is obtained at $k \approx 12\,800$, higher than for model $\mathcal{M}_1$. However, by accounting for both the possible specifications, the innovative drug is still cost-effective for a range of values of k.

by effect of the implications of the model in which $\rho = 1$. The CEAC is also slightly lower in the averaged model, with a value of 0.652 for $k = 25\,000$. On the other hand, the EVPI is quite similar, indicating that overall the remaining uncertainty on the parameters is not very large. □

3.7 Advanced issues in cost-effectiveness analysis

3.7.1 Including a risk aversion parameter in the net benefit

The previous analysis is based on the use of the monetary net benefit to describe the utility of the decision-maker. As suggested earlier, this presupposes a form of risk-neutrality on the part of the decision-maker. However, this assumption might not be reasonable. In fact, in most cases it could be argued that the decision-maker is rather risk-averse, i.e. they need to limit the uncertainty about the optimality of the decision process.

The above analysis can be extended to consider a more general form for the utility function, to include explicitly the possibility that the decision-maker is risk-averse (Baio and Dawid, 2011). This has obvious implications on the level and quality of the evidence used to reach the decision.

We consider again the model presented in §3.3.1, but instead of the simple linear utility function of equation (3.5) used so far, we now define a more complex form

$$u(b,r) = \frac{1}{r}\left[1 - \exp(-rb)\right],\qquad\qquad (3.18)$$

where $r > 0$ represents a parameter of *risk aversion* (Raiffa, 1968) — the higher the value of r, the more risk-averse the decision-maker — and $b := ke-c$ denotes the monetary net benefit.

Now, in line with the analysis of §3.4, the quantity that we should investigate for PSA of uncertainty in the parameters, the known-distribution utility of equation (3.7), has the more complex form

$$
\begin{aligned}
U(\theta^t) &= \int \frac{1}{r}\left[1 - \exp(-rb)\right] p(b \mid \theta^t)\, db \\
&= \frac{1}{r}\left[1 - M_{B|\theta^t}(-r)\right]
\end{aligned}
$$

where $M_{B|\theta^t}(-r) := \mathrm{E}[\exp(-rB)]$ is the moment generating function of the random quantity B with respect to the distribution $p(b \mid \theta^t)$, evaluated at the point $-r$. Notice that in this case the utility function is no longer linear in (e,c) and will be in general not straightforward to compute analytically. However, it will typically be available via a simulation approach, such as the MCMC procedure we are using here.

Example (continued)

The function CEriskav in the package BCEA can be used to perform the analysis including risk aversion in the utility function. The inputs to this function are a bcea object (i.e. the output of an economic analysis obtained using the bcea function) and a vector of values for the risk aversion parameter r. The commands

```
r <- c(0.000000000001,0.00000001,0.000000025,0.000000050)
cr <- CEriskav(m,r)
```

execute the analysis, saving the output in an object cr. The results can be plotted by using the specialised function

```
plot(cr,k=m$k)
```

which takes as inputs the object cr and the vector of possible values for the willingness-to-pay parameter. In this case, we use those selected in the object m (i.e. a grid of values between 0 and 50 000, as defined earlier).

Figure 3.11 shows the expected incremental benefit EIB for various values of r and as a function of k, and highlights the important effect on the overall decision process of including the risk propensity of the decision-maker.

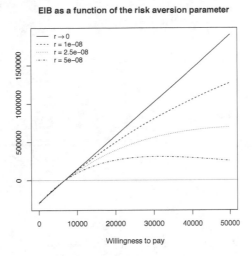

EIB as a function of the risk aversion parameter

FIGURE 3.11

Analysis of the expected incremental benefit including a parameter of risk aversion. For each value of the willingness-to-pay parameter k, we present the EIB for different choices of the risk aversion parameter r. Upon varying this, the shape of the EIB changes significantly, and becomes increasingly non-linear.

When $r \to 0$ the decision-maker is risk-neutral, and EIB is identical with that based on the monetary net benefit utility function. Notice, however, the break even point (i.e. the value of k for which the new drug becomes the best option, producing a positive EIB) may in general vary upon changing the value of r. Moreover, as r increases from 0, EIB becomes increasingly non linear.

Figure 3.12 shows the analysis of the EVPI as a function of k and r; again, for $r \to 0$ we retrieve the same analysis of Figure 3.7. When the decision-maker's risk-aversion is taken into account, the expected value of information becomes generally lower since with the new utility function larger values of k are associated with less uncertainty. Notice that this is not always the case and in fact in some situations the results will be reversed (with utilities accounting for risk-aversion bringing to higher values of the EVPI for higher k).

In any case, while the analysis of the EVPI is appropriately sensitive to the choice of r, it is possible to prove with standard probability calculus that using the utility function of equation (3.18) the CEAC is independent of the value of

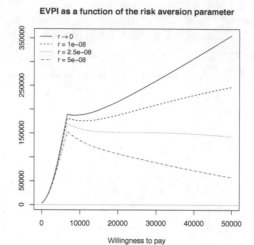

FIGURE 3.12

PSA by means of the EVPI, accounting for risk aversion. Different choices of r imply a different shape for the EVPI. In particular, the break even point (i.e. the point corresponding to the value of k where the optimal decision changes from the status quo to vaccination) changes for the four scenarios analysed. This is due to the different decision-maker's attitude to risk, as specified by r.

r. This is essentially because r is a multiplicative scale parameter and as such, while it does modify the shape of the distributions of IB (and therefore the expected values used to compute the EVPI), it does not affect the probability that IB is positive. Consequently, irrespective of the risk propensity of the decision-maker, if PSA is performed using the CEAC the results are the same (and identical with that depicted in Figure 3.4). Again, this feature is not ideal, as we would expect different decision-makers with different attitude towards risk to arrive at different results.   □

3.7.2   Expected value of information for mixed strategies

In real practice it is rarely the case that a treatment proves to be cost-effective over the entire population, therefore justifying the fact that the market includes more than one therapeutic option for the same condition. As suggested earlier, this is mainly due to the fact that implementing an intervention is typically associated with some risks such as irreversibility of investments, thus justifying the fact that the decision-maker might want to temporise, in order to have more reliable evidence on which to base the final decision. Moreover, the market usually takes some time to "adjust" to the new configuration generated by the innovative intervention just introduced.

Consequently, we are often faced with the problem of balancing the optimal decision (i.e. implementing the most cost-effective treatment, while discontinuing the other options) with the constraints represented by the fact that the market shares of the other interventions already available to the decision-maker to manage the same condition (i.e. all t different from the option that maximises the expected utility) cannot be all set directly to zero (see Baio and Russo, 2009 for a more detailed discussion).

Under this constraint, the *actual* expected utility in the overall population can be computed as the mixture

$$\bar{\mathcal{U}} = \sum_t q_t \mathcal{U}^t = q_0 \mathcal{U}^0 + q_1 \mathcal{U}^1, \tag{3.19}$$

assuming that q_0 and $q_1 = (1 - q_0)$ are the market share that will be obtained in the future by the two treatments considered. Notice that the situation can be easily extended to the case where, say, T alternatives are present on the market; in this case, we would have a vector of market shares $\mathbf{q} = (q_0, q_1, \ldots, q_{T-1})$, with $q_{T-1} = 1 - (q_0 + \ldots + q_{T-2})$.

The quantity $\bar{\mathcal{U}}$ can be compared with the "optimal" expected utility $\mathcal{U}^*$ to evaluate the market loss induced by the less than perfect resource allocation.

Example (continued)

The function mixedAn in the package bcea is used to performed the analysis of the mixed strategy. First we need to define the vector of market shares for all the treatment in analysis. Assuming in the running example that the standard drug will remain market leader with $2/3$ of the shares, we do this by typing the command mkt.shares <- c(.66,.33). This is one of the inputs required by the function.

Then, we launch the command ma <- mixedAn(m,mkt.shares), which uses the output of the original economic analysis saved in the object m and computes (3.19). The result of the analysis can be then displayed graphically by typing the command plot(ma).

Figure 3.13 shows the expected value of information computed assuming the combination of market shares $(q_0, q_1) = (0.67, 0.33)$. In other words, we assume that even after the cost-effectiveness analysis developed above shows that the new chemotherapy drug is the optimal choice for values of $k \geq 6\,700$ the two drugs are simultaneously present on the market.

The analysis of Figure 3.13 is incremental with respect to the "ideal" situation where for each k the option with the highest overall utility is chosen (which, in this example, amounts to setting $q_1 = 0$ for $k < £6\,700$ where $t = 0$ is the most cost-effective option, and $q_1 = 1$ for $k \geq £6\,700$), represented by the solid bold line. The light line represent the mixed expected utility obtained in correspondence of the combination of the two alternatives.

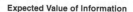

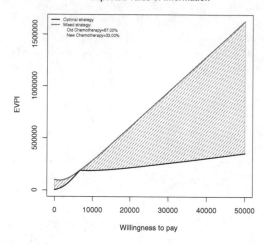

FIGURE 3.13
Analysis of the expected value of information for the mixed strategy and for different values of the market shares.

As is possible to see, in the area where $t = 0$ is the preferred option, leaving both drugs on the market does not produce a large increase in the expected value of information. This makes intuitive sense, as the old treatment maintains most of the market shares and the EVPI is lower anyway.

When k gets closer to the break-even point, uncertainty as to whether either of the treatments is cost-effective is at its maximum. Consequently, using the mixed strategy produces a lower loss, which is eventually 0 at the break-even point (as one can see, the two curves coincide for $k \approx £6\,700$).

After the break-even point, $t = 1$ becomes the best option. Consequently, the difference between the optimal strategy and the mixed option becomes increasingly larger. This makes sense because the preferred option is consumed with lower market shares.   □

In general, the mixed strategy analysis can be used in several different ways, according to the perspective of the subject affected by this uncertainty: for example, the pharmaceutical company proposing the new treatment at the predicted market share (q_1); or the pharmaceutical company distributing the already available treatment, less cost-effective with respect to the new one, at the corresponding market share $q_0 = (1 - q_1)$. In both cases, the value of the uncertainty could be used in order to: (a) establish the amount of investment for clinical research that would be cost-effective to reduce the uncertainty about the optimal decision; (b) determine the proposed reimbursed retail price, in terms of reduction of the proposed reimbursed price; or (c) represent the payback value from the pharmaceutical company to the regional provider.

This last case could be considered after the marketing of the new product, since it depends on the market shares really associated with all the alternative options.

4

Bayesian analysis in practice

4.1 Introduction

As discussed in Chapter 2, if it is possible to sample from the full conditional distributions, Gibbs sampling algorithms can be programmed in a relatively easy way. However, in most practical situations, the required conditional distributions are not analytically tractable and therefore it is necessary to approximate them (e.g. by means of algorithms such as Metropolis-Hastings or slice sampling) before Gibbs sampling can be performed.

The most popular software that allows the semi-automatisation of the MCMC procedures is BUGS, and particularly its MS Windows incarnations WinBUGS (Spiegelhalter et al., 2002) and OpenBUGS (Lunn et al., 2009), whose widespread use has arguably contributed to the establishment of applied Bayesian statistics in the last twenty years.

The acronym BUGS stands for *Bayesian analysis Using Gibbs Sampling* and the program essentially consists of two main parts. The first is a *parser*, which inspects the set of declarations provided by the user to define the statistical model (in terms of data and parameter distributions and, possibly, other deterministic relationships among the variables in the problem). In particular, the parser codifies the statistical model in terms of the corresponding DAG, trying to make use of the conditional independence relationships implied by the model assumed by the user. These generally simplify the computations, since the full conditional distribution for any (set of) node(s) only involves a local computation on the graph. Thus, only a small portion of the whole model needs to be considered at any given time (Lunn et al., 2009).

The second part is an expert system that is used to deduce the form of the full conditional distributions generated by the problem. When possible, BUGS tries to exploit conjugacy to speed up the process; when this is not feasible, suitable complementary sampling algorithms are applied together with the Gibbs sampling to obtain the required MCMC estimation.

While both BUGS and WinBUGS can run as stand-alone software, in recent years several programs have been written to interface them with standard statistical software such as R, Matlab, Stata or SAS, which makes the process of data analysis easier (we discuss this aspect later).

Despite their wide success, WinBUGS or BUGS are not the only possible alternative. An increasingly popular, albeit very similar language that offers a few advantages is JAGS (*Just Another Gibbs Sampler*, Plummer, 2010). One of these is that JAGS is an open-source project written in C++, which means it is effectively platform independent. Since every operating system has a C++ compiler and standard library, JAGS can be run natively under MS Windows, Unix/Linux or Mac. In contrast, BUGS and WinBUGS are coded in Component Pascal, a relatively obscure language implemented in a particularly low-level environment, known as the *Black Box Component Builder*, with compiler available only for MS Windows (although the latest release of OpenBUGS does run under Linux).

Moreover, it is generally easier to interface JAGS with existing software written in C or C++, e.g. linear algebra routines for matrix operations, or the R package for statistical functions math (which can be used to produce samples from probability distributions). Similarly to WinBUGS, JAGS can be interfaced with R by means of suitable libraries.

In the next sections we describe the main characteristics of the JAGS language and its implementation from within an R session to perform Bayesian analysis in practice. However, since the differences between BUGS and JAGS code are generally minimal, it is possible to use nearly the same commands to run a Bayesian analysis in BUGS or WinBUGS.

Interesting references (including many worked examples) on Bayesian analysis with MCMC implemented in either of these software packages are Congdon (2001, 2003, 2010), Spiegelhalter et al. (2004), Woodworth (2004), Carlin and Louis (2009), Ntzoufras (2009), Jackman (2009) and Kruschke (2011).

4.2   Software configuration

We consider a computer configuration that includes the current versions of R (which is downloadable from http://cran.r-project.org). In addition, one of either JAGS (available from http://mcmc-jags.sourceforge.net) or BUGS (http://www.mrc-bsu.cam.ac.uk/bugs/overview/contents.shtml; WinBUGS can be obtained from the same website, while OpenBUGS is available at http://www.openbugs.info) needs to be installed on the machine. Guidance on the installation under different operating systems is available from the respective websites. All examples considered here use R 2.14 and JAGS 3.2.0.

Finally, we need a suitable library to interface R with the MCMC software. For JAGS, we use R2jags (Su and Yajima, 2010), while for BUGS/WinBUGS it is possible to use packages such as R2WinBUGS (Sturtz et al., 2005) or BRugs (Thomas et al., 2012). These libraries allow the user to perform the analysis from within R. For example, to install R2jags we type the R commmand[1]

---

[1]As suggested earlier, we could alternatively install and use WinBUGS. In this case, in

```
install.packages("R2jags")
```

The code to describe the statistical model to be run needs to be saved in an external text file, and suitable commands launch either JAGS or BUGS/WinBUGS in background. Once the MCMC run is finished, the simulations become available in the R session where the user is able to post-process them to complete the Bayesian analysis.

4.3 An example of analysis in JAGS/BUGS

Consider again Laplace's analysis of §2.4.1. Using a Uniform prior on the probability that a newborn is female, the analysis is straightforward and in fact does not require MCMC estimation. However, we start with this very simple example to show how the procedure works.

The statistical analysis via MCMC estimation is performed through several steps:

- specifiying and validating the model;

- loading the data;

- assigning initial values;

- performing the Gibbs sampling simulations;

- checking convergence;

- analysing the output.

First of all, we load the required package with the command

```
library(R2jags)
```

R is now ready to interface with JAGS.

4.3.1 Model specification

The next step we need to perform is to code the modelling assumptions in a text file that can be passed to JAGS as input. This can be done in any text editor (e.g. Notepad in MS Windows, or gedit in Unix/Linux).

Every JAGS/BUGS code begins with the instruction model followed by a curly bracket "{" and ends with the enclosing bracket "}". All the declarations

---

R we should type the commands install.packages("R2WinBUGS"). To install packages from remote repositories, it is necessary to have an active internet connection.

regarding the data model, the prior distributions and other possible deterministic relationships among the variables need to be included between the two curly brackets.

In this case, the model is very simple and can be coded in the following way.

```
model {
    theta ~ dunif(0,1)
    y ~ dbin(theta,n)
}
```

In the BUGS/JAGS language, probability distributions are described by suitable strings including the prefix d (for "distribution"), followed by an abbreviation of the name. Thus, in this case the syntax dbin indicates the Binomial distribution with parameters defined as the probability of "success" (theta) and the sample size (n). A detailed account of all the distributions supported by JAGS/BUGS can be found in the software manuals.

Since BUGS/JAGS are *declarative* languages, the actual order in which the commands are written is not important. Thus, it is possible to specify the data model before the prior distribution for a parameter, although the former depends on the latter.

Probabilistic assignments are identified by the symbol ~, much as in standard statistical terminology. Deterministic relationships must be defined using the symbol <-. Using one symbol instead of the other, e.g. by typing theta <- dunif(0,1), will cause JAGS or BUGS/WinBUGS to stop with a syntax error.

Once the model has been translated in the BUGS/JAGS language, we need to save it to a text file. The easiest option is to use a .txt format, e.g. ModelLaplace.txt. At this point, we need to go back to the R session to set up the call to JAGS and run the analysis.

4.3.2   Pre-processing in R

Before we can run JAGS we generally need some pre-processing to be performed in R. In general, a Bayesian model will be based on observed data, which need to be passed to JAGS as input. Larger datasets will have larger size for the implied DAG of the model, thus requiring a longer time to process.

In this simple case, the observed data are the total number of babies ($n = 493\,527$) and the number of female births ($y = 241\,945$). We can load these values in R by means of the simple commands

```
y <- 241945
n <- 493527
```

In order to interface with the JAGS/BUGS program, we need to put these variables in a data list, which we do in R by typing

```
data <- list("y","n")
```

Alternatively, it is possible to define the data object as a "named list" of the form data <- list(y=y,n=n). The main difference between the two formats is that the former defines a list of *names* for the variables to be used by JAGS, while the latter specifically defines the objects themselves. Thus using the named list format one can directly access the *value* (in addition to the name) of the data, when working in R.

Obviously, in more general cases, the dataset to be used will be more complex and perhaps will be imported in R from a spreadsheet or a database manager (in this case, the library foreign can be installed to help). However, the underlying logic is the same and all the variables that are observed and part of the model need to be included in the data list.

The next step is to define the initial values for the simulation. Both JAGS and BUGS/WinBUGS can automatically generate initial values for the unobserved variables in the model: to do so, it is sufficient to set inits <- NULL.

However, this might create some problems when using vague specifications, for which incompatible initial values might be generated (e.g. a negative value for a variance)[2]. Moreover, when the initial values are generated automatically, every chain is started from the same pseudo-random point, which has obvious problems for the analysis of the $\hat{R}$ statistic (2.19). Consequently, whenever possible it is best to pass some suitable initial values to the procedure. This can be obtained in two different ways.

The easiest is to create another list in which deterministic values are assigned to all unobserved random variables. In the current example, this can be obtained for instance by defining the list:

```
inits <- list(theta=.5)
```

Alternatively, a better solution is to create a function that generates initial values from a suitable probability distribution suggested by the user and according to the problem at hand. In R this can be obtained by using the following code[3]

```
inits <- function(){list(theta=runif(1))}
```

Since in the present model the node theta represents a probability, it has to be bounded in the interval [0, 1] and therefore selecting a random value from a Uniform(0,1)[4] distribution will certainly provide a sensible initial value.

---

[2]Technically, this problem only occurs with BUGS/WinBUGS, which selects the initial values as random draws from the prior distribution. Conversely, JAGS uses some suitable "central values" (e.g. the mean, median or mode), thus avoiding the issue entirely.

[3]In R, the syntax function() defines a function with no arguments.

[4]In R, the general command to generate random draws from the Uniform distribution is runif(n,lower,upper), where n is the number of values to simulate, and lower and upper specify the interval in which the distribution is defined. By default, these are set to 0 and 1, respectively. Thus the syntax runif(n) draws n values from a Uniform(0,1) distribution. Similarly, for the Normal distribution the syntax is rnorm(n,mean,sd), with mean and sd representing the mean and the standard deviation of the required distribution. Since the default values are 0 and 1, respectively, the syntax rnorm(n) draws n values from the standard Normal distribution.

If the model considers more than just one variable to be initialised, it is easy to extend the definition of the function `inits` by including in the list comma-separated suitable values for the other variables. For example, if the model included a further unobserved random node mu represented by a vector of size 10 and associated with a Normal distribution, then a suitable code would be:

```
inits <- function(){list=(theta=runif(1),mu=rnorm(10))}
```

In this case, R would generate 10 values from a standard Normal distribution that would be used by JAGS to initialise the node mu.

The last part of the pre-processing operation involves the definition of an R object which contains the variables to be monitored in the MCMC procedure. In the present case, the only parameter in the model is the probability of a female birth, so this can be done by typing

```
params <- "theta"
```

In more realistic cases in which the number of nodes to monitor is greater than one, it is easy to extend this syntax to generate a *collection* of nodes into the object params. For instance, if we also needed to monitor the node mu, we could type

```
params <- c("theta","mu")
```

Obviously, there is no need to use the names above to identify the data list, the initial values and the parameters to monitor. Any string accepted by R represents a valid name.

Finally, it is useful to define an R variable including the path to the model file, for instance in MS Windows something like

```
filein <- "C:/JagsModels/ModelLaplace.txt"
```

or in Unix/Linux

```
filein <- "/home/gianluca/JagsModels/ModelLaplace.txt"
```

4.3.3   Launching JAGS from R

At this point, we are ready to finally launch JAGS to execute the MCMC procedure and obtain the sample of simulations from the posterior distribution. This can be done by calling the function jags in the package R2jags. An example of the syntax required is the following[5]

```
model <- jags(data=data,inits=inits,parameters.to.save=params,
              model.file=filein,n.chains=2,n.iter=10000,
              n.burnin=4500,n.thin=1,DIC=TRUE)
```

---

[5]When using WinBUGS and R2WinBUGS, the command is slightly modified to launch the bugs function. Most of the options are the same and we refer to the library help for the differences.

The function `jags` creates an object `model` and takes several inputs. The first three are the data list, the initial values and the parameters to be monitored. As mentioned earlier, it is possible to use different names for these R objects, as long as they are correctly referenced within the function.

Then we need to specify the model file, i.e. the `txt` file which contains the specification of the model. In this case we have already created the variable `filein` which directs R to the physical position in which the file is stored.

The next inputs specify the number of chains to be run, the burn-in and whether to use thinning (cfr. §2.4.5). The total number of iterations stored for the analysis is equal to `n.chains`×(`n.iter`−`n.burnin`)/`n.thin`. In the present example, we consider 9500 simulations with a burn-in of 4500 for 2 chains and with thinning equal to 1 (which means that every simulation is considered, or no thinning at all). Thus, the number of iterations used for the MC analysis is $2 \times (9500 - 4500)/1 = 10000$.

Finally, the option `DIC=TRUE` instructs JAGS to monitor the model deviance, and to compute and report the value of the DIC, defined in equation (3.16). Notice that for models in which no random quantity is observed, this option is not available, since JAGS cannot compute the model deviance in that case (and therefore it is necessary to set `DIC=FALSE` in the inputs of the call to the `jags` function).

There are other possible options to be used in the call to the `jags` function (e.g. the possibility of selecting the working directory), but we do not normally need to set them and in general the default values are acceptable. Typing `help(jags)` in the R terminal shows the full description of the function and its usage.

When the function `jags` is launched, R responds with the following output

```
Compiling model graph
    Resolving undeclared variables
    Allocating nodes
    Graph Size: 5

Initializing model
```

JAGS first compiles the model to derive the corresponding DAG; then it tries to resolve undeclared variables, if any are present. If it fails to do so because of an incorrect specification of the model, an error message will be generated. While, as remarked earlier, the variables can be entered in the JAGS code in no particular order, the compilation step is quicker if the top-level parameters are defined first (i.e. parameters before the observable variables and hyper-parameters before the parameters).

If everything has worked until this point, JAGS allocates the nodes in the graph and calculates the size of the DAG. This is computed by counting the number of nodes involved in the model. In this example, the nodes are `y`, `n`, `theta`. Moreover, JAGS creates a node for each function or arithmetic expression used in the model; in this case the two extremes of the Uniform distribution associated with θ are defined internally as two additional nodes, bringing the total size of the DAG to 5. As mentioned earlier, realistic models are associated with a much larger size.

Finally, JAGS initialises the model, depending on the way in which the user has specified the variable inits. If it is set to NULL, it automatically generates random initial values. Alternatively, it either uses the list of deterministic values, or the user-defined function that generates random draws from specific distributions.

After initialisation, the model is run. A text bar shows the progression through the required simulations; a running series of asterisks * is printed and the counter is incremented while the iterations are generated. When the counter reaches 100%, R takes over JAGS and the user regains control over the session.

At this point, R contains an object model of the class rjags, which contains the MCMC output and can be used to perform the Bayesian analysis.

4.3.4 Checking convergence and post-processing in R

Objects in the class rjags have a specific method print which can be used to produce a summary of the distributions obtained by the MCMC procedure. By typing

```
print(model,digits=3,intervals=c(0.025, 0.975))
```

we ask R to show a summary table for the object model. In particular, we specify the options requesting that all figures are shown with 3 decimal places and that the 2.5– and 97.5–th percentiles are shown. Of course, it is possible to modify this to include more decimal places or more/different quantiles of the distributions (by default, also the 25–, 50– and 75–th percentiles are displayed). In response to this command, R produces the following table.

```
Inference for Bugs model at "ModelLaplace.txt", fit using jags,
 2 chains, each with 9500 iterations (first 4500 discarded)
 n.sims = 10000 iterations saved

          mu.vect sd.vect   2.5%  97.5%  Rhat n.eff
theta       0.490   0.001  0.489  0.492 1.001 10000
deviance   14.543   1.370 13.562 18.527 1.001 10000

For each parameter, n.eff is a crude measure of effective sample size,
and Rhat is the potential scale reduction factor
(at convergence, Rhat=1).

DIC info (using the rule, pD = var(deviance)/2)
pD = 0.9 and DIC = 15.5
DIC is an estimate of expected predictive error
(lower deviance is better).
```

The summary table shows the values of the mean, standard deviations and the required percentiles from the posterior distributions for each node monitored. Moreover, the statistics used to check convergence (cfr. §2.4.5) are also shown. In this simple case, convergence is pretty obvious (as the model is conjugate) — the Gelman–Rubin statistic (2.19) has a value which is lower than 1.1 and the number of effective replications (2.20) is identical with the number of iterations monitored. In addition to the node theta, JAGS monitors the model deviance, since we specified the option DIC=TRUE, and gives some basic information on how to use it.

Additional methods to check convergence are implemented in the package rjags (which is automatically loaded with R2jags). In order to use these methods, we first need to format the object model as an mcmc structure, which is done creating a new object m with the command m <- as.mcmc(model).

Typing raftery.diag(m) produces the following input.

```
[[1]]
Quantile (q) = 0.025
Accuracy (r) = +/- 0.005
Probability (s) = 0.95
```

	Burn-in (M)	Total (N)	Lower bound (Nmin)	Dependence factor (I)
deviance	2	3866	3746	1.030
theta	2	3620	3746	0.966

```
[[2]]
Quantile (q) = 0.025
Accuracy (r) = +/- 0.005
Probability (s) = 0.95
```

	Burn-in (M)	Total (N)	Lower bound (Nmin)	Dependence factor (I)
deviance	2	3620	3746	0.966
theta	2	3866	3746	1.030

By default, the Raftery-Lewis diagnostics estimates the number of iterations required to estimate q, the 2.5% quantile of the posterior distribution, with an accuracy (tolerance) r of ±0.005 and a probability s of 0.95 of being within that tolerance. These parameters can of course be varied to any quantile, tolerance and probability level.

For each chain (in the output, the notation [[1]] indicates the first chain, [[2]] indicates the second, and so on), R reports the number of iterations N and the burn-in M necessary to satisfy the specified conditions. The quantity Nmin indicates the minimum number of iterations that need to be used to perform the estimation of N, while the dependence factor I can be interpreted as the proportional increase in the number of iterations attributable to serial dependence. Dependence factors exceeding 5 are considered to be high and suggestive of problems; these may be due to influential starting values, large correlations between parameters, or poor mixing in general.

In this case, because the model is extremely simple and uses conjugacy, the number of burn-in iterations required is only 2. An MC estimation based on just over 3600 iterations after convergence would be able to estimate with very large precision even the extreme quantiles of the posterior distribution of the main variable (theta). The very low value of the dependence factor indicates that there are no problems with autocorrelation.

Another useful indicator of convergence is provided by the *Monte Carlo error*. This can be obtained by typing summary(m), which produces the following result.

```
Iterations = 1:5000
Thinning interval = 1
Number of chains = 2
Sample size per chain = 5000

1. Empirical mean and standard deviation for each variable,
   plus standard error of the mean:

             Mean        SD  Naive SE Time-series SE
deviance 14.5430 1.3696383 1.370e-02      1.322e-02
theta     0.4902 0.0007053 7.053e-06      7.575e-06

2. Quantiles for each variable:

             2.5%     25%     50%     75%   97.5%
deviance 13.5616 13.6664 14.0208 14.8743 18.5265
theta     0.4889  0.4898  0.4902  0.4907  0.4916
```

The value of the "Naive Standard Error" is computed as the ratio of the posterior standard deviation for a given node to the number of simulations and can be then used to express the MC error (rather than posterior uncertainty). The Time-series SE adjusts the Naive SE for autocorrelation. Of course, lower values indicate better convergence. In this case, both estimates are very low, which again confirms the findings discussed above.

The results produced by the MCMC procedure are in line with the closed-form analysis shown in §2.4.1: the posterior mean of the probability of a female birth is 0.490 and a 95% credible interval is computed as $[0.489; 0.492]$, which suggests that $\theta < 0.5$ as concluded by Laplace.

The object model contains several elements that can be listed by typing names(model), which produces the following output

```
[1] "model"           "BUGSoutput"      "parameters.to.save"
[4] "model.file"      "n.iter"          "DIC"
```

Each element of the object can be accessed with the usual R syntax. For instance, typing model$model produces the R output

```
JAGS model:

model {
y ~ dbin(theta,n)
theta ~ dunif(0,1)
}
```

```
Fully observed variables:
 n y
```

The element `model$BUGSoutput` contains the actual MCMC output and can be made accessible from within the R session with the command[6]

```
attach.bugs(model$BUGSoutput)
```

After this is launched, it is possible to work directly on the simulated arrays for each variable[7]. For instance, it is easy to produce a graphical representation of the posterior distribution of θ, by typing `hist(theta)`, which produces the result shown in Figure 4.1.

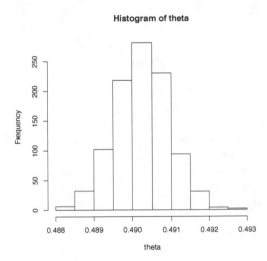

FIGURE 4.1
A histogram from the posterior distribution of the probability of a female birth, θ, generated by the MCMC simulations.

Convergence of each node can also be inspected graphically, producing a traceplot using the object `model$BUGSoutput$sims.array`, which contains an array of dimension $\left[\left(\frac{s-b}{t}\right), c, p\right]$, where: s is the total number of simulations performed; b is the number of simulations discarded in the burn-in; t represents the thinning; c is the number of chains; and p is the number of parameters monitored.

---

[6]When using `WinBUGS` and `R2WinBUGS`, the command is modified to `attach.bugs(model)`.

[7]The MCMC simulation process increments by one dimension the size of each variable: for instance, a node representing a scalar becomes a vector (S MCMC iterations), a node originally defined as a vector becomes a matrix (S MCMC iterations for each of the K elements of the vector) and so on.

In the current example the dimension of `sims.array` is $(500, 2, 2)$ and the traceplot can be obtained with the following commands:

```
plot(model$BUGSoutput$sims.array[1:500,1,"theta"], t="l",
    col="blue", xlab="Iteration", ylab="",
    ylim=range(model$BUGSoutput$sims.array[1:500,1:2,"theta"]))
points(model$BUGSoutput$sims.array[1:500,2,"theta"], t="l", col="red")
```

The command `plot` is used to draw the traceplot for the first chain. The relevant positions in the three-dimensional array are chosen by selecting:

- the elements from 1 to 500 along the first dimension of the array (i.e. all the 500 simulations);

- the value 1 for the second dimension (which instructs R to use the first chain);

- the element identified by the name `"theta"` along the third dimension (which contains the saved parameters).

Similarly, the syntax `[1:500,2,"theta"]` selects all the simulations for the node `theta` for the second chain.[8]

The option `ylim=range(model$BUGSoutput$sims.array[,1:2,"theta"])` is used to choose the range on the $y-$axis, which spans from the minimum to the maximum value across the two chains for the simulated values for `theta`.

Finally, the command `points` is used to add the traceplot for the second chain to that for the first one. If we used the command `plot` again, R would clear the graph and only show the second chain (i.e. the last requested by the user).

As mentioned earlier, in this case convergence is quite certain and the mixing for the two chains is clearly satisfactory, as Figure 4.2 shows.

4.4   Logical nodes

Often, a statistical model contains a set of *logical* variables, whose definition is based on a deterministic relationship. The classical example is given by the linear regression model, in which the observable variable is defined as $y \sim$ Normal(μ, σ^2) and the mean is defined in terms of a deterministic relationship with a set of regressors, e.g. in the form $\mu = \alpha + \mathbf{X}\beta$.

In general, despite the fact that the relationship used to define them is deterministic, in a statistical model logical nodes are functions of random

---

[8]Technically, the syntax `1:500` is redundant: since there really is no selection and all the units are included, to identify all the elements along the first dimension of the array `model$BUGSoutput$sims.array` it is sufficient to leave the first slot in the square brackets empty, e.g. `[,1,"theta"]`.

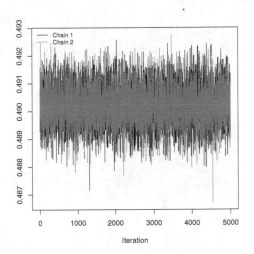

FIGURE 4.2
A traceplot for the node `theta` produced by the R code using the simulations
stored in the object generated by JAGS.

nodes (e.g. the regression coefficients) and therefore are random quantities
themselves, often representing the focus of the analysis.

Consider again Laplace's analysis and suppose that we want to estimate
the posterior probability that $\theta < 0.5$. It is easy to include this by simply
augmenting the existing model with the command

```
p.50 <- step(theta - 0.5)
```

by means of the assignment of the logical node `p.50`. In this case we use the
built-in BUGS/JAGS function `step`, generally defined as:

$$\text{step(x)} = \begin{cases} 1 & \text{if } x \geq 0 \\ 0 & \text{otherwise.} \end{cases}$$

Again, we refer to the software manual for a list of all the logical functions
supported by BUGS/JAGS.

In the current example, at each MCMC iteration, the node `p.50` takes
value 1 if the probability of a female birth is simulated to be greater than
or equal to the cut-off point of 0.5, and 0 otherwise. Thus, using the set of
iterations obtained after convergence, the node `p.50` estimates the posterior
probability that female births are more or equally likely than male births.

Notice how in the BUGS/JAGS language the functional relationship between
two nodes has to be written using the symbol `<-` (instead of the `=`, typically
used in algebra). As is often the case with programming languages, BUGS/JAGS

distinguish between the situation in which two variables have the same value
(which is identified by the symbol =) and that in which the value of a variable
is computed, i.e. when the symbol <- is assigned. Using the wrong notation
generates a syntax error when compiling the model.

We can modify the JAGS/BUGS code to include the node p.50:

```
model {
    theta ~ dunif(0,1)
    y ~ dbin(theta,n)
    p.50 <- step(theta-0.5)
}
```

and save the new model in a file `ModelLaplace2.txt`. We can now rerun the
analysis calling JAGS by typing

```
params <- c("theta","p.50")
model2 <- jags(data=data,inits=inits,parameters.to.save=params,
               model.file="ModelLaplace2.txt",n.chains=2,
               n.iter=5000,n.burnin=4500,n.thin=1,DIC=TRUE)
```

This time we specify the model file directly in the call to the function jags,
implicitly assuming that the file `ModelLaplace2.txt` is saved in the working
directory, i.e. the directory currently in use by R. If this were not the case, we
could specify the complete path to the file within the function.

Also, since the new model does not contain extra unobserved random quantities, there is no need to modify the function inits (the node p.50 is a deterministic quantity and as such it *cannot* be initialised). However, before we
launch the function jags, we need to modify the variable params since now
we also want to monitor the new node p.50.

After the model has run, it is possible to see the summary results, by typing
`print(model2,digits=3,intervals=c(0.025, 0.975))`, which produces the
following output

```
Inference for Bugs model at "ModelLaplace2.txt", fit using jags,
 2 chains, each with 5000 iterations (first 4500 discarded)
 n.sims = 1000 iterations saved
          mu.vect sd.vect  2.5%  97.5% Rhat n.eff
p.50         0.00   0.000 0.000  0.000 1.000    1
theta        0.49   0.001 0.489  0.492 1.000 1000
deviance    14.60   1.403 13.562 18.614 1.002 1000

For each parameter, n.eff is a crude measure of effective sample size,
and Rhat is the potential scale reduction factor
(at convergence, Rhat=1).

DIC info (using the rule, pD = var(deviance)/2)
pD = 1.0 and DIC = 15.6
DIC is an estimate of expected predictive error
(lower deviance is better).
```

Much as in Laplace's original analysis, the chance that θ exceeds the threshold of 0.5 is estimated to be negligible. Notice also that because there is effectively no variability in the simulations for the node p.50 (i.e. all the simulated values are equal to 0), the number of effective replications is 1. We can still rely on the Gelman–Rubin statistic $\hat{R}$ to check convergence (which is clearly reached, in this case).

4.5 For loops and node transformations

Another important aspect of many statistical models is the fact that we generally have a sample of (conditionally) independent observations from a common distribution. In programming terms, this is can be coded by using for loops.

Consider again the final example of Chapter 2, in which we specified two different forms of linear regression analysis. The first model, $\mathcal{M}_1$, was:

$$\left.\begin{array}{l} y_i \sim \text{Normal}(\mu_i, \sigma^2) \\ \mu_i = \alpha + \beta X_i \end{array}\right\} \text{ for } i = 1, \ldots, N$$

$$\alpha, \beta \sim \text{Normal}(0, h^2) \quad \text{independently,}$$

$$\log(\sigma) \sim \text{Uniform}(-k, k)$$

for some observed response y and covariate X, and for some large values h and k, say for definiteness $h = 100$ and $k = 5000$.

The natural way to express this model in JAGS/BUGS language is to make use of a for loop to replicate the distributional assumptions for each value i. This can be programmed quite easily, using a syntax that is very similar to that of R:

```
model {
    for (i in 1:N) {
        y[i] ~ dnorm(mu[i],tau)
        mu[i] <- alpha + beta*X[i]
    }
    prec <- 1/pow(h,2)
    alpha ~ dnorm(0,prec)
    beta ~ dnorm(0,prec)
    lsigma ~ dunif(-k,k)
    tau <- pow(exp(lsigma),-2)
}
```

The definition of the loop is quite intuitive: first, we set the range of the incrementing index i using the syntax for (i in 1:N). Notice that JAGS/BUGS require a space between the index of the loop and the word in, and then another space between in and the starting point (1, in this case). Failure to follow this spacing convention will cause a syntax error.

The loop is delimited by two curly brackets and every instruction contained within the two brackets is replicated for N times. Quantities that vary with each value of the index i need to be defined using the syntax `variable[index]`, e.g. in this case `y[i]`.

Notice that not all the quantities defined inside a loop depend on the index i. For example, the regression coefficients `alpha` and `beta` are scalars that do not vary with the different data points. Hence they are not associated with the `[i]` notation. However, all nodes in the left-hand side of a statement inside a loop must be defined as a function of the index. For example, if we coded

```
model {
    for (i in 1:N) {
        y[i] ~ dnorm(mu[i],tau)
        mu <- alpha + beta*X[i]
        ...
```

then for each value of i the node `mu` would be overwritten, because the expression `alpha + beta*X[i]` assumes different values upon varying i. This would generate an error of multiple definition for `mu`.

Similarly, to include an expression depending on some indexes outside a loop, e.g.

```
model {
    for (i in 1:N) {
        y[i] ~ dnorm(mu[i],tau)
    }
    mu[i] <- alpha + beta*X[i]
    ...
```

will cause JAGS/BUGS to stop with an error message.

The necessity to define the linear predictor in a separate line of the code is a peculiarity of BUGS/WinBUGS and it is one of the fundamental differences with JAGS. In fact, in JAGS it is possible to embed deterministic nodes inside other expressions, for instance using a more compact notation

```
    for (i in 1:N) {
        y[i] ~ dnorm(alpha + beta*X[i],tau)
    }
```

Another noteworthy aspect of the code is the fact that in JAGS/BUGS the Normal distribution is indexed by the mean and the precision (i.e. the reciprocal of the variance, cfr. §2.4.5). In this case, we indicate the precision of the observed data `y[i]` with the node `tau`, while the node `prec`, explicitly defined as the reciprocal of h^2, is the precision of the regression coefficients.

The reason for this unusual convention is that parameterising the Normal distribution in terms of the precision simplifies the use of the conjugate

Gamma prior (cfr. Table 2.3). This was particularly relevant in the first releases of BUGS, when computational speed was still an important issue even for simple models, but the notation has stuck and JAGS follows it too.

In general terms, one can still set a prior distribution on the precision scale. In fact, a minimally informative conjugate Gamma(ϵ, ϵ) prior (with ϵ an arbitrarily small positive number, e.g. 0.0001) is often assumed by default. Gelman (2006) discusses the implications of this choice, suggesting that in the limit of $\epsilon \to 0$ this prior gives an improper posterior density. Especially for hierarchical models (cfr. §5.3), inferences become very sensitive to the choice of ϵ, limiting the robustness of this prior distribution.

Consequently, even to encode vague knowledge, it is often advisable to specify the prior on (transformations of) the variance or the standard deviation, as we do in the current example. If this modelling strategy is followed, it is necessary to include some suitable conditions in the model statements, to link the node which has the status of random quantity to the precision.

For example, in the above code we first specify a prior distribution for lsigma (which indicates the logarithm of the standard deviation). Then we need to create a deterministic relationship between lsigma and tau, which otherwise would be undefined, generating an error message. This can be done by using the logical functions pow and exp to code the mathematical relationships $\tau := 1/\sigma^2 = \sigma^{-2} = \exp(\log(\sigma))^{-2}$.

The model is completed with the specification of the Normal prior distributions for the nodes alpha and beta and the final result is saved in the file modelNormal.txt.

Assuming that the data for (y, X) are already loaded in the workspace, we can run the analysis by using the following R code:

```
N <- length(y)
h <- 100
k <- 5000
dataJags <- list("N","y","X","h","k")
filein <- "modelNormal.txt"
params <- c("alpha","beta","sigma")
inits <- function(){
   list(alpha=rnorm(1),beta=rnorm(1),lsigma=rnorm(1))
}
m <- jags(dataJags, inits, params, model.file=filein,
   n.chains=2,n.iter=10000,n.burnin=9500,n.thin=1,DIC=TRUE)
print(m,digits=3,intervals=c(0.025, 0.975))
```

First we define the constant variables N, h and k which identify respectively the number of observations, the standard deviation of the regression coefficients and the scale of the prior Uniform distribution.

The need to create a separate node to define the upper bound of a loop is another source of major difference between BUGS/WinBUGS and JAGS. In fact, JAGS language allows the user to query the size of vectors or arrays that are supplied in the data file. Consequently, in this case we could modify the first few lines of the model file as:

```
model {
    for (i in 1:length(y)) {
        y[i] ~ dnorm(mu[i],tau)
        ...
```

so that we would not need to define the node N, or to include it in the data list.

We then define the data list including all the observed quantities, which in this case are y, X, k and N, and create a string variable with the path to the model file.

The next steps select the parameters to be monitored in the MCMC procedure (in this case we choose the two regression coefficients and the population standard deviation) and then define the inits function. In this example, we instruct R to draw the initial values from a standard Normal distribution. This choice is reasonable given the distributional assumptions and random draws from a standard Normal are effectively certain to produce valid starting points for these variables.

Finally, we run the function jags for 2 chains with 10000 iterations, a burn-in of 9500 and no thinning, to produce the output

```
Inference for Bugs model at "modelNormal.txt", fit using jags,
 2 chains, each with 10000 iterations (first 9500 discarded)
 n.sims = 1000 iterations saved
             mu.vect sd.vect      2.5%      97.5%  Rhat n.eff
alpha     -2292.936  88.791 -2499.307  -2135.080 1.145    37
beta        142.025   2.286   138.052    147.426 1.140    38
sigma       455.821   9.823   436.836    474.993 1.027   220
deviance 16817.813    4.648 16808.253  16826.721 1.097   160

For each parameter, n.eff is a crude measure of effective sample size,
and Rhat is the potential scale reduction factor
(at convergence, Rhat=1).

DIC info (using the rule, pD = var(deviance)/2)
pD = 10.7 and DIC = 16828.6
DIC is an estimate of expected predictive error
(lower deviance is better).
```

As suggested in Chapter 2, convergence is poor for this model, as confirmed by the diagnostics in the summary table. Centering the covariate would help with this aspect of the modelling.

4.5.1   Blocking to improve convergence

Sometimes an alternative way to improve convergence is to use "*blocking*" for (some of) the parameters. With this terminology we indicate the situation where instead of having several univariate nodes to represent the parameters in a model, we use a joint multivariate distribution to model them. This generally speeds up the mixing of the chains because the Gibbs sampling steps will use the full conditional of the whole block of parameters, rather than several univariate full conditionals.

In the current example, we could for instance specify a prior joint distribution on the intercept and slope of the regression model. The new formulation of the model is:

```
model {
    for (i in 1:N) {
        y[i] ~ dnorm(mu[i],tau)
        mu[i] <- alpha + beta*X[i]
    }
    # Blocking of coefficients
    coef[1:2] ~ dmnorm(m[1:2],P[1:2,1:2])
    alpha <- coef[1]
    beta <- coef[2]

    lsigma ~ dunif(-k,k)
    sigma <- exp(lsigma)
    tau <- pow(sigma,-2)
}
```

which we save in a separate file named `modelNormalBlocking.txt`.

Most of the code is unchanged except for the inclusion of a new node `coef` which is associated with a multivariate Normal distribution. JAGS/BUGS syntax requires the user to specify the dimension of the multivariate node, which in this case is done by adding `[1:2]` to the name of the variable. This tells JAGS/BUGS that the node `coef` is a vector with two components. In the next line of the code, the first element is then associated to the intercept `alpha`, while the second is the slope `beta`.

The syntax `dmnorm` indicates the multivariate Normal distribution, which simply extends the univariate case to a mean vector `m` with two elements (one for the first and the other for the second component of the variable `coef`) and a 2-by-2 precision matrix, `P`.

In the current example, we need to define these before we can run the model. For consistency with the unblocked model, we select suitable values so that the prior on the regression coefficients is minimally informative, for instance:

$$m = \begin{pmatrix} 0 \\ 0 \end{pmatrix} \quad \text{and} \quad P = \frac{1}{h^2} \begin{pmatrix} 1 & 0 \\ 0 & 1 \end{pmatrix}.$$

These assumptions imply that we are assuming that the two elements of the node `coef` are uncorrelated, since the precision matrix is diagonal.

We can program this by typing in R the following code:

```
m <- c(0,0)
prec <- (1/h^2)*diag(2)
```

and we can finally run the blocked model using the following instructions:

```
dataJags <- list("m","P","N","y","X","k")
filein <- "modelNormalBlocking.txt"
params <- c("alpha","beta","sigma")
inits <- function(){
  list(lsigma=rnorm(1),coef=rnorm(2,0,1))
}
n.iter <- 10000
n.burnin <- 9500
n.thin <- floor((n.iter-n.burnin)/500)
m.blc <- jags(dataJags, inits, params, model.file=filein,
  n.chains=2, n.iter=10000, n.burnin=9500, n.thin=1,DIC=TRUE)
print(m.blc,digits=3,intervals=c(0.025, 0.975))
```

— notice that for simplicity we choose to initialise the node `coef` using two independent draws from a standard Normal distribution). After JAGS has run, we obtain the following summary table.

```
Inference for Bugs model at "modelNormalBlocking.txt", fit using jags,
 2 chains, each with 10000 iterations (first 9500 discarded)
 n.sims = 1000 iterations saved
            mu.vect sd.vect      2.5%      97.5% Rhat n.eff
alpha     -2315.383 172.176 -2660.840 -1980.158 1.002  1000
beta        142.618   4.419   133.818   151.468 1.001  1000
sigma       456.191   9.490   439.227   474.994 1.005  1000
deviance 16817.213   8.408 16802.892 16836.169 1.001  1000

For each parameter, n.eff is a crude measure of effective sample size,
and Rhat is the potential scale reduction factor
(at convergence, Rhat=1).

DIC info (using the rule, pD = var(deviance)/2)
pD = 33.8 and DIC = 16850.9
DIC is an estimate of expected predictive error
(lower deviance is better).
```

As is possible to see, convergence is improved massively and is reached satisfactorily for all the nodes involved in the model.

4.6 Predictive distributions

Often, in a Bayesian model it is required to compute the predictive distribution (2.11), for some of the random quantities involved. This is extremely easy to programme in JAGS/BUGS and can be achieved by simply extending the standard model introducing an additional node.

Consider again the regression model above, but assume that this time we want to include in the analysis the prediction for a yet unobserved replication of y. For example, we might be interested in the value of the response variable for the next individual, which we indicate with y^* and consider as exchangeable with the observed vector $\mathbf{y} = (y_1, \ldots, y_N)$.

In line with the discussion of §2.3.1, this means that the we assume a common functional form for the distributions of y^* and $\mathbf{y}$. Moreover, when estimating the distribution of y^*, we consider the *current* uncertainty on the parameters, i.e. that provided by the posterior distribution $p(\boldsymbol{\theta} \mid \mathbf{y})$.

Suppose that in model $\mathcal{M}_1$ above, the response y represents the birth weight in grams of a newborn, while the covariate X is the gestational age, i.e. the estimated number of weeks since conception. The objective of the model is to predict the birth weight of the next baby, given the current uncertainty on the parameters $\boldsymbol{\theta} = (\alpha, \beta, \sigma)$ and some specific value of X, say X^*.

We can obtain this by simply extending the model as:

```
model {
    for (i in 1:N) {
        y[i] ~ dnorm(mu[i],tau)
        mu[i] <- alpha + beta*X[i]
    }
    alpha ~ dunif(-k,k)
    beta ~ dunif(-k,k)
    lsigma ~ dunif(-k,k)
    tau <- pow(exp(lsigma),-2)
    sigma <- exp(lsigma)

    # Predictive distribution
    y.star ~ dnorm(mu.star,tau)
    mu.star <- alpha + beta*X.star
}
```

which we save in a new file modelNormal2.txt.

Most of the code remains unchanged. The only new parts involve the inclusion of a new node y.star to which we associate a Normal distribution that is characterised by the same precision as the observed data $\mathbf{y}$. Similarly, the mean mu.star has the same functional form as the mean mu, with the only difference being in the specific value of the covariate X.star.

Figure 4.3 shows the DAG of this model. In particular, the solid arrows indicate the assumed model, i.e. the data generating process that we are considering. Conversely, the dashed arrows show the process by which the observed evidence is used to update uncertainty on the unobserved random quantities. Thus, the inference on the node y^* is performed conditionally on the current level of information, i.e. after observing $(\mathbf{y}, \mathbf{X}, X^*)$.

Suppose that the assumed value for X^* is 28 weeks. This might be an actual observed variable (e.g. if we want to predict the birth weight of a new baby, knowing that the mother has gone into labour at exactly that estimated

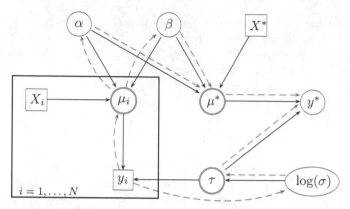

FIGURE 4.3
Graphical representation of the model in terms of a DAG. Nodes enclosed in circles or ovals represent unobserved random quantities. Squared nodes indicate observed data. Double-rounded nodes indicate logical variables, defined as deterministic functions of other nodes in the graph. The box around the nodes indexed by i means that the same structure is repeated for N times. The solid arrows indicate the structure assumed for the data generating process, while the dashed arrows indicate the posterior updating obtained by means of the Bayesian procedure.

gestational age), or a hypothetical value (e.g. if the doctor wants to plan different care strategies for a mother who has not gone into labour yet).

We can then run the model using the following code.

```
X.star <- 28
dataJags2 <- list("N","y","X","k","X.star")
filein <- "modelNormal2.txt"
params2 <- c("alpha","beta","sigma","y.star")
inits <- function(){
    list(alpha=rnorm(1),beta=rnorm(1),
        lsigma=rnorm(1),y.star=runif(1,0,6000))
}
m2 <- jags(dataJags2, inits, params2, model.file=filein,
    n.chains=2,n.iter=50000,n.burnin=4500,n.thin=91,DIC=TRUE)
print(m2,digits=3,intervals=c(0.025, 0.975))
```

After we have set the value for the new estimated gestational age X.star, we redefine the data list to include this node as well. Then we redefine the name of the model file to point JAGS towards the new specification and the object containing the parameters to be monitored so that the predictive distribution of y.star is included.

The next modification to the previous R code is in the `inits` function, where we set an initial value also for the node y.star. Technically, this is not strictly necessary; in fact, JAGS/BUGS will estimate the predictive distribution effectively using a simple MC approach (such as the one discussed in §2.4.3) using for each iteration the current value of the relevant parameters and thus there is no issue of convergence. However, it is generally a good idea to provide reasonable starting values for any non-observed random quantity, and in this case we do so by providing a value from a Uniform distribution in the interval $[0; 6000]$.

Finally, we run the `jags` function for 50000 iterations using the first 9500 for the burn-in and thinning of 81. This implies that the simulations saved to produce the posterior inference are 1000. The results are saved in the object m2 which is then printed to give the following output.

```
Inference for Bugs model at "modelNormal2.txt", fit using jags,
 2 chains, each with 50000 iterations (first 9500 discarded),
 n.thin = 81, n.sims = 1000 iterations saved
            mu.vect sd.vect      2.5%      97.5%  Rhat n.eff
alpha    -2343.609 169.118 -2667.398 -2023.663 1.000  1000
beta       143.319   4.333   135.147   151.706 1.000  1000
sigma      455.764   9.928   436.599   476.001 1.002  1000
y.star    1677.155 460.291   743.366  2565.684 1.000  1000
deviance 16815.939   8.107 16802.916 16833.459 1.000  1000

For each parameter, n.eff is a crude measure of effective sample size,
and Rhat is the potential scale reduction factor
(at convergence, Rhat=1).

DIC info (using the rule, pD = var(deviance)/2)
pD = 32.9 and DIC = 16848.8
DIC is an estimate of expected predictive error
(lower deviance is better).
```

From the summary table, we can conclude that convergence is sufficiently reached. The nodes `alpha`, `beta` and `sigma` have low values for the Gelman–Rubin statistics and the effective sample size is identical with the number of iterations saved. The predicted birth weight for the next baby born at a gestational age of 28 weeks is 1.68kg. As is reasonable, the precision of this estimation is not very high, as confirmed by the large credible interval associated with it.

4.6.1 Predictive distributions as missing values

An alternative way of estimating a predictive distribution is to consider the future observation to be estimated y^* as a *missing completely at random* (sometimes referred to as MCAR) data point in the series of the observed **y**. The reasoning underlying this strategy is the same as used before: we assume that $\mathbf{y} = (y_1, \ldots, y_N)$ are exchangeable with the $(N+1)$-th observable value $y^* := y_{(N+1)}$.

In a sense, this is more straightforward to code, since it does not require the definition of an additional node in the model. The way in which JAGS/BUGS handle this is to include an extra data point coded as NA (not available, i.e. missing) for the (now) last observation.

In R we can code this using the following command:

```
y <- c(y,NA)
```

which augments the original data vector for the variable y by one additional unit, whose value is NA.

If we are using BUGS/WinBUGS convention, we now need to also update the value of the sample size, stored in the variable N. This can be done by re-running the command N <- length(y), which will now increment the original value by virtue of the inclusion of the $(N+1)$−th missing data point. On the contrary, if we were using JAGS convention, we could just leave this part of the model program unchanged and let the command for (i in 1:length(y)) in the model file deal with the different sample size automatically.

Either way, we can still use the original model file stored as modelNormal.txt to run the analysis. The analysis is then executed by using the following R commands.

```
X <- c(X,28)
filein <- "modelNormal.txt"
params3 <- c("alpha","beta","sigma","y")
inits <- function(){
   list(alpha=rnorm(1),beta=rnorm(1),lsigma=rnorm(1),
        y=c(rep(NA,(N-1)),rnorm(1)))
}
m3 <- jags(dataJags, inits, params3, model.file=filein,
   n.chains=2,n.iter=50000,n.burnin=9500,n.thin=81,DIC=TRUE)
```

First, we need to augment the covariate vector to also include the value for $X^* = 28$. The data list is identical with that used for the analysis where no predictive distribution is considered. This makes sense, as the two model codes are the same and so are the data required to run. Thus there is no need to redefine it here.

The R variable containing the parameters to be monitored, however, is different from the two previous versions considered above. In the first model it did not make sense to monitor y because it was *entirely* observed, while in the second we added the extra unobserved node y.star to estimate the predictive distribution. In this case, we need to add the node y, which is only *partially* observed, to the parameters list.

Similar reasoning applies for the initial values: in the first two models, y cannot be initialised because it is an entirely observed variable and therefore JAGS/BUGS do not need a starting point for the simulation. However, in this case y contains unknown values and therefore it is necessary to initialise it.

Much as in the model for the predictive distribution developed above by using the extra node y.star, it is possible to let JAGS/BUGS generate the starting point by not including y in the inits function. However, if we want to provide an initial value ourselves, we need to bear in mind that the first $(N-1)$ cases are completely observed (recall that we have incremented by one unit the original value of N) and therefore cannot be given initial values. Thus, we define the relevant element in the `inits` function by a collection of $(N-1)$ NAs, created by the R command `rep(NA,(N-1))`, plus one single draw from a standard Normal distribution. In this way, only the missing point (which is the last one in the data list) is initialised.

When we select a large number of parameters to be monitored, the call to the `print` function is likely to produce an output that is difficult to read, because of the large number of rows of the ensuing table. For instance, using the parameters list defined in the object `params3` above, the command `print(m3,digits=3,intervals=c(0.025, 0.975))` would produce a table including the summary statistics from the posterior distribution of the entire vector y. Of course, because they are directly observed, the first $(N-1)$ values would not be very interesting; on the contrary, the interest would only be on the regression coefficients, the population standard deviation and the N−th element of the vector y.

To overcome this problem, there are two possible ways: the first one is to include the whole vector y in the parameters list and directly access the summary table through the object `m3$BUGSoutput$summary`. By default, the number of rows of the summary table is p, the total number of parameters monitored, including the single elements of vector parameters (so that if in a given model we decided to monitor a scalar and a vector of 9 elements, p would be equal to 10). On the other hand, the columns of the summary table contain the statistics for the mean, the standard deviation, the 2.5%, 25%, 50%, 75% and 97.5%–th percentiles of the posterior distributions, the Gelman–Rubin statistic and the effective sample size, i.e. 9 in total.

Thus, using for instance the code

```
m3$BUGSoutput$summary[c(1:4,N+4),c(1:3,7:9)]
```

selects the rows 1, 2, 3, 4 and $(N+4)$ and the columns 1, 2, 3, 7, 8, and 9 of the overall summary table to produce the following output:

```
              mean      sd       2.5%      97.5%  Rhat  n.eff
alpha    -2335.986  165.296 -2660.064  -2015.828 1.010   410
beta       143.144    4.245   134.955    151.506 1.009   440
deviance 16816.337    7.940 16802.072  16833.521 1.008   510
sigma      456.108   10.109   436.892    475.670 1.000  1000
y[1116]   1694.942  462.886   807.411   2605.153 1.000  1000
```

(here the index 1116 is equal to N). Other relevant information, as for instance the values for the DIC, can be accessed by querying the object `m3$BUGSoutput`, e.g. by typing `m3$BUGSoutput$DIC`.

Alternatively, we can select in the parameters list only the elements of the vector y on which we want to make inference. In the present case, this can be done for example by typing

```
params4 <- c("alpha","beta","sigma","y[1116]")
```

and running the model with the usual call to the function jags. The command

```
print(m3,digits=3,intervals=c(0.025, 0.975))
```

would now produce a table with the four monitored nodes (plus the deviance if the option DIC=TRUE is selected), such as the following.

```
Inference for Bugs model at "modelNormal.txt", fit using jags,
 2 chains, each with 50000 iterations (first 9500 discarded),
 n.thin = 81, n.sims = 1000 iterations saved
            mu.vect  sd.vect      2.5%      97.5% Rhat n.eff
alpha     -2335.986 165.296 -2660.064  -2015.828 1.010   410
beta        143.144   4.245   134.955    151.506 1.009   440
sigma       456.108  10.109   436.892    475.670 1.000  1000
y[1116]    1694.942 462.886   807.411   2605.153 1.000  1000
deviance 16816.337   7.940 16802.072  16833.521 1.008   510

For each parameter, n.eff is a crude measure of effective sample size,
and Rhat is the potential scale reduction factor
(at convergence, Rhat=1).

DIC info (using the rule, pD = var(deviance)/2)
pD = 31.5 and DIC = 16847.8
DIC is an estimate of expected predictive error
(lower deviance is better).
```

As is possible to see from the summary table, the results are in line with the previous analysis, although perhaps a slightly higher level of autocorrelation is present in this model.

4.7   Modelling the cost-effectiveness of a new chemotherapy drug in R/JAGS

Consider again the cost-effectiveness analysis of a new chemotherapy drug, discussed in §3.3. The simple modelling assumptions presented earlier are programmed with the following code:

```
model {
# Observed data on side effects and ambulatory care
    for (s in 1:N.studies) {
        se[s] ~ dbin(pi[1],n[s])
        amb[s] ~ dbin(gamma,se[s])
    }

# Prior distributions
    pi[1] ~ dbeta(a.pi,b.pi)
```

```
      pi[2] <- pi[1]*rho
      rho ~ dnorm(m.rho,tau.rho)
      gamma ~ dbeta(a.gamma,b.gamma)
      c.amb ~ dlnorm(m.amb,tau.amb)
      c.hosp ~ dlnorm(m.hosp,tau.hosp)

  # Predictive distributions on the clinical outcomes
      for (t in 1:2) {
          SE[t] ~ dbin(pi[t],N)
          A[t] ~ dbin(gamma,SE[t])
          H[t] <- SE[t] - A[t]
      }
  }
```

which we save in the file `modelChemo.txt`. In order to run it, we need to provide apposite values for the hyper-parameters defining the distributions. Notice that in JAGS/BUGS it is not possible to associate an element of a vector or of a matrix with the index 0. Thus we use the notation `pi[1]` and `pi[2]` to indicate respectively π_0 and π_1 (and similarly for SE, A and H).

In the code, we first model the observed data provided by `N.studies` ($=$ 5) published studies. For each study, we have information on `se`, the number of patients showing side effects out of the `n` investigated, and on `amb`, the number of patients with side effects requiring only ambulatory care. We use this information to update the uncertainty about the parameters π_0 and γ.

As suggested earlier, sometimes it is possible to encode prior information in suitable probability distributions by taking advantage of their mathematical properties. For instance, given the assumed values of the mean m and standard deviation s for a Beta random variable, it is possible to derive α and β by using (2.15).

We can write a simple R function that takes the values for (m, s) as input and returns the values of the parameters (α, β) that characterise the Beta distribution that we use to represent the prior uncertainty.

```
betaPar <- function(m,s){
  a <- m*((m*(1-m)/s^2)-1)
  b <- (1-m)*((m*(1-m)/s^2)-1)
  list(a=a,b=b)
}
```

The function `betaPar` computes the parameters, which we indicate as a and b, and then stores them in a list, from which they can be accessed by using the `object$element` notation.

For instance, for the parameter π_0 representing the probability that a patient treated with the standard drug experiences side effects we assumed vague prior knowledge. This can be translated in a mean of 0.5 and a large variance, e.g. 0.125. The code

```
m.pi <- .5
s.pi <- sqrt(.125)
a.pi <- betaPar(m.pi,s.pi)$a
b.pi <- betaPar(m.pi,s.pi)$b
```

computes the variables `a.pi` = 0.5 and `b.pi` = 0.5 (cfr. Table 3.1), which represent the parameters of the Beta distribution that we associate with π_0. We can visualise the implied prior distribution by typing in R:

```
pi0 <- rbeta(10000,a.pi,b.pi)
hist(pi0,main="",xlab=expression(pi[0]))
```

which draws 10000 values from a Beta distribution with parameters `a.pi` and `b.pi` and then produces a histogram of the sample, shown in Figure 4.4. The option `main=""` instructs R to put no title on the graph, while `xlab=expression(pi[0])` writes the symbol π_0 as the x-axis label).

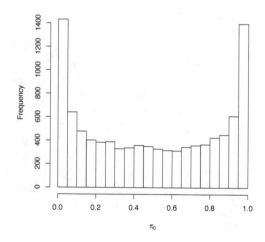

FIGURE 4.4

A minimally informative Beta prior distribution for the parameter π_0.

We can use the function `betaPar` to derive the distributions of the parameters that are associated with a Beta prior. Notice however, that this is not the only possible way of doing so. For instance, Christensen et al. (2011) describe a method to derive the parameters of a Beta distribution when information on its quantiles is known. A further alternative way of formalising the hyper-parameters is by thinking of α as the number of successes observed in $(\alpha + \beta)$ hypothetical trials performed before the current data are made available (Spiegelhalter et al., 2004).

We can use similar reasoning to deal with the random quantities that are assumed to be associated with a logNormal distribution (e.g. the cost for ambulatory care). By definition of the logNormal density, if m and s are the population mean and standard deviation on the natural scale, then the parameters on the logarithmic scale μ and σ^2 can be derived as:

$$\mu = \log(m) - \frac{1}{2}\log\left(1 + \frac{s^2}{m^2}\right) \quad \text{and} \quad \sigma^2 = \log\left(1 + \frac{s^2}{m^2}\right).$$

We can code this in the function `lognPar`, defined in R as:

```
lognPar <- function(m,s) {
  s2 <- s^2
  mulog <- log(m)-0.5*log(1+s2/m^2)
  s2log <- log(1+(s2/m^2))
  sigmalog <- sqrt(s2log)
  list(mulog=mulog,sigmalog=sigmalog)
}
```

Suitable values for all the remaining hyper-parameters can be derived by running the following code in R, in which we also load the values of the observed data.

```
m.gamma <- .5
s.gamma <- sqrt(.125)
a.gamma <- betaPar(m.gamma,s.gamma)$a
b.gamma <- betaPar(m.gamma,s.gamma)$b

m.rho <- 0.8
s.rho <- 0.2
tau.rho <- 1/s.rho^2

mu.amb <- 120
sd.amb <- 20
m.amb <- lognPar(mu.amb,sd.amb)$mulog
s.amb <- lognPar(mu.amb,sd.amb)$sigmalog
tau.amb <- 1/s.amb^2

mu.hosp <- 5500
sd.hosp <- 980
m.hosp <- lognPar(mu.hosp,sd.hosp)$mulog
s.hosp <- lognPar(mu.hosp,sd.hosp)$sigmalog
tau.hosp <- 1/s.hosp^2

# Observed data
c.drug <- c(110,520)        # unit cost of drugs
N <- 1000                   # population size
```

```
n <- c(32,29,24,33,23)        # sample size for the studies
se <- c(9,3,7,4,9)            # data on side effects
amb <- c(5,2,3,2,5)           # data on ambulatory care
N.studies <- length(n)        # number of studies
```

Notice that in the JAGS/BUGS language the logNormal distribution is also defined in terms of the precision. Thus after computing the value of the standard deviation on the logarithmic scale by means of the function lognPar, we also compute the precision by squaring its reciprocal. This is the actual hyperparameter that is then passed to the jags function, which is called typing:

```
dataJags <- list("a.pi","b.pi","a.gamma","b.gamma",
                 "m.amb","tau.amb","m.hosp","tau.hosp",
                 "m.rho","tau.rho","N","se","amb","N.studies")
filein <- "modelChemo.txt"
params <- c("pi","gamma","c.amb","c.hosp","rho","SE","A","H")
inits <- function(){
    list(pi=c(runif(1),NA),gamma=runif(1),c.amb=rlnorm(1),
        c.hosp=rlnorm(1),rho=runif(1))
}
chemo <- jags(dataJags, inits, params, model.file=filein,
    n.chains=2,n.iter=20000,n.burnin=9500,n.thin=42,DIC=FALSE)
print(chemo,digits=3,intervals=c(0.025, 0.975))
attach.bugs(chemo$BUGSoutput)
```

First we define the data list, by including all the hyper-parameters, and the parameters to be monitored. As for the initial values we note that only the first element of the vector parameter pi is in fact a random quantity, as the second one is defined as a deterministic function. Therefore, we need to initialise it using a collection of values, the second of which is NA in the function inits. Technically, the unobserved variables SE and A need to be initialised as well, but we let JAGS take care of this by not including them in the inits function.

The results of the model are summarised in the following table.

```
Inference for Bugs model at "model.txt", fit using jags,
 2 chains, each with 20000 iterations (first 9500 discarded),
 n.thin = 42, n.sims = 500 iterations saved
```

	mu.vect	sd.vect	2.5%	97.5%	Rhat	n.eff
A[1]	120.278	28.949	65.475	178.525	1.007	450
A[2]	97.156	34.562	39.950	178.525	1.015	120
H[1]	106.972	26.349	60.000	162.050	1.001	500
H[2]	86.248	31.483	34.475	152.050	1.007	200
SE[1]	227.250	35.123	160.000	292.000	1.001	500
SE[2]	183.404	54.985	84.475	297.000	1.017	299
c.amb	119.451	19.873	85.263	161.277	1.007	500
c.hosp	5481.781	987.622	3867.277	7655.766	1.007	200
gamma	0.530	0.090	0.339	0.689	1.001	500
pi[1]	0.228	0.033	0.161	0.295	1.002	500
pi[2]	0.183	0.054	0.088	0.300	1.024	284
rho	0.801	0.198	0.405	1.177	1.029	178

```
deviance   40.326   2.014   38.389   45.351 1.005   500
```

For each parameter, n.eff is a crude measure of effective sample size, and Rhat is the potential scale reduction factor (at convergence, Rhat=1).

DIC info (using the rule, pD = var(deviance)/2)
pD = 2.0 and DIC = 42.4
DIC is an estimate of expected predictive error
(lower deviance is better).

Convergence seems to be reached satisfactorily as all the nodes are associated with low values of the Gelman–Rubin statistic, as well as with relatively large values of the effective sample size. Consequently, we can use the simulations produced by JAGS to perform the health economic analysis.

First we make them available to the R workspace attaching the elements of the object chemo, which is done by typing `attach.bugs(chemo$BUGSoutput)`. Then we compute the relevant measures of cost and effectiveness using the code:

```
e <- c <- matrix(NA,chemo$BUGSoutput$n.sims,2)
e <- N - SE
for (t in 1:2) {
    c[,t] <- c.drug[t]*(N-SE[,t]) +
            (c.amb+c.drug[t])*A[,t] +
            (c.hosp+c.drug[t])*H[,t]
}
```

Notice that we need to allocate the new variables e and c in the R memory. To do so, we define each of them as a matrix of size `chemo$BUGSoutput$n.sims` (the number of simulations saved) by 2 (the number of interventions considered). Initially, we fill these matrices with NAs, which are then overwritten by the commands following in the code.

At this point, we are ready to load and run the function bcea to perform the analysis shown throughout Chapter 3.

4.7.1 Programming the analysis of the EVPPI

As suggested in §3.5.3, the results of the MCMC simulation model can be also used to perform an analysis of the EVPPI for some of the parameters.

In general, it is convenient to save in a separate variable the simulated values for the parameter which is the object of the EVPPI, in this case ρ. Since the elements of the object chemo$BUGSoutput have been made available to the R session earlier, it is sufficient to type `rho.sim <- rho` to do so.

In addition, it is necessary to slightly modify the model code, since we now want to separate the two layers of parameter uncertainty. The first one accounts for the imprecise knowledge about the distribution of ρ, estimated by the values in the vector rho.sim and derived by the posterior analysis conducted earlier on the "complete" model. The second layer of uncertainty considers the variation in the remaining parameters given each simulated value for ρ.

Thus, we delete the fourth line rho ~ dnorm(m.rho,tau.rho) of the original model code and save the resulting file (shown below) as modelEVPPI.txt.

```
    model {
# Observed data on side effects and ambulatory care
    for (s in 1:N.studies) {
        se[s] ~ dbin(pi[1],n[s])
        amb[s] ~ dbin(gamma,se[s])
    }

# Prior distributions
    pi[1] ~ dbeta(a.pi,b.pi)
    pi[2] <- pi[1]*rho
    gamma ~ dbeta(a.gamma,b.gamma)
    c.amb ~ dlnorm(m.amb,tau.amb)
    c.hosp ~ dlnorm(m.hosp,tau.hosp)

# Predictive distributions on the clinical outcomes
    for (t in 1:2) {
        SE[t] ~ dbin(pi[t],N)
        A[t] ~ dbin(gamma,SE[t])
        H[t] <- SE[t] - A[t]
    }
}
```

The following R code can be then used to perform the EVPPI analysis.

```
K <- length(m$k)
Ustar.phi <- matrix(NA,chemo$BUGSoutput$n.sims,K)

#1. Loops on all the simulated values of rho.sim
for (i in 1:chemo$BUGSoutput$n.sims) {
    rho <- rho.sim[i]

#2. Prepares the data, parameters and inits and runs the MCMC
    dataJags <- list("a.pi","b.pi","a.gamma","b.gamma","m.amb",
                    "tau.amb","m.hosp","tau.hosp","rho","N",
                    "se","amb","n","N.studies")
    filein <- "modelEVPPI.txt"
    params <- c("pi","gamma","c.amb","c.hosp","SE","A","H")
    inits <- NULL
    n.iter <- 10000
    n.burnin <- 9750
    n.thin <- floor((n.iter-n.burnin)/250)
    chemo.evppi <- jags(dataJags, inits, params, model.file=filein,
        n.chains=2, n.iter, n.burnin, n.thin, DIC=TRUE)
```

```
#3. Performs the economic analysis given the simulations
#    for all the other parameters, conditionally on rho
     attach.bugs(chemo.evppi$BUGSoutput)
     e.temp <- c.temp <- matrix(NA,chemo$BUGSoutput$n.sims,2)
     e.temp <- N - SE
     for (t in 1:2) {
         c.temp[,t] <- c.drug[t]*(N-SE[,t]) +
                       (c.amb+c.drug[t])*A[,t] +
                       (c.hosp+c.drug[t])*H[,t]
     }
     m.evppi <- bcea(e=e.temp,c=c.temp,ref=2,interventions=treats,
                     Kmax=50000,Ktable=25000)

#4. Computes the maximum expected utility for the current iteration
#    and for each value of k
     Ustar.phi[i,] <- apply(m.evppi$Ustar,2,mean)
     rm(m.evppi); detach.bugs()
}

#5. Computes the average value of the maximum expected utility
#    for each value of k
Vstar.phi <- apply(Ustar.phi,2,mean)

#6. Computes the EVPPI for each value of k
Umax <- apply(apply(m$U,c(2,3),mean),1,max)
EVPPI <- Vstar.phi - Umax
```

First, we define the object Ustar.phi, in which we will store the conditional "known distribution" utilities $U^*(\phi)$, as a matrix with the number of rows equal to chemo$BUGSoutput$n.sims (the number n_{out} of simulations generated for the original health economic analysis, in this case 500), and as many columns as the number of points in the grid used for the willingness to pay k (cfr. §3.3.3). We assume that the output of the function bcea has been saved in the object m and we indicate this number as K (= 501 in this case).

Next, we programme a loop in which the following instructions are executed. First the i−th value of rho.sim is assigned to the variable rho. This ensures that the health economic analysis will be performed conditionally on the parameter of interest ($\phi = \rho$), but accounting for the uncertainty in all the other parameters ψ.

While the data list is unchanged, the model file variable is modified to direct JAGS to the new one and the parameters list is modified to exclude rho, which in the current case is not a random quantity. For simplicity, we let JAGS initialise the chains by setting the function inits to the value NULL.

Once the number of iterations, burn-in and thinning are defined, we can call the function jags, which runs the model and saves the results in the object chemo.evppi. The simulations can be then used to rerun the health economic analysis: we attach the MCMC simulations to the R session, compute the measures of cost and effectiveness just as we have done for the "complete" analysis and save the output of bcea in the object m.evppi.

At each iteration, bcea computes the known-distribution utility in the element m.evppi$Ustar. This is a matrix with the number of rows equal to chemo.evppi$BUGSoutput$n.sims = n_{inn} (i.e. the number of simulations obtained in the MCMC procedure just run; 500 in this case), and K columns.

The uncertainty about ψ is integrated out by computing the average, which can be done using the R command apply(m.evppi$Ustar,2,mean). The result is a vector of K maximum expected utilities $U^*(\phi)$, which we save in the i−th row of the matrix Ustar.phi.

At this point, we remove the object m.evppi, detach the simulations from the R workspace and move to the next value of rho.sim. When the loop is completed, we can proceed to integrate the second level of uncertainty, i.e. that related to the imperfect knowledge of ϕ.

This is done by computing the average value of the variable Ustar.phi. The R code apply(Ustar.phi,2,mean) applies the function mean to each row of Ustar.phi and the result is saved in the vector Vstar.phi, which has length K.

The final task before we can compute the EVPPI is to obtain for each k the overall maximum expected utility $\mathcal{U}^*$. The element m$U, included in the object m contains the utility $U(\theta^t)$ calculated for each of the n_{out} simulations, each of the K values of the willingness to pay and each of the n_{int} interventions. Thus, in this case, it is an array of dimensions (500, 501, 2).

In order to obtain $\mathcal{U}^*$, we first compute the mean over the simulations (i.e. the first dimension of m$U) and then compute the maximum value using the R syntax apply(apply(m$U,c(2,3),mean),1,max), to produce a vector Umax of K elements. The difference between Vstar.phi and Umax gives the EVPPI, which can then be plotted against the values of k to produce Figure 3.8.

4.7.2 Programming probabilistic sensitivity analysis to structural uncertainty

In line with the discussion of §3.6, we need to define a new model file in which the parameter ρ is set to 1, with no uncertainty. To do so, we can actually re-use the file modelEVPPI.txt, in which the node rho was already considered as a fixed quantity.

However, we now need to pass the correct value of 1 to JAGS. This can be done using the following R code.

```
detach.bugs()
rho <- 1
dataJags <- list("a.pi","b.pi","a.gamma","b.gamma","m.amb",
                 "tau.amb","m.hosp","tau.hosp","rho","N",
                 "se","amb","n","N.studies")
filein <- "modelEVPPI.txt"
params <- c("pi","gamma","c.amb","c.hosp","SE","A","H")
inits <- function(){
    SE=rbinom(2,N,.2)
    list(pi=c(runif(1),NA),gamma=runif(1),c.amb=rlnorm(1),
```

```
                 c.hosp=rlnorm(1),SE=SE,A=rbinom(2,SE,.2))
}
n.iter <- 20000
n.burnin <- 9500
n.thin <- floor((n.iter-n.burnin)/250)
chemo2 <- jags(dataJags, inits, params, model.file=filein,
        n.chains=2, n.iter, n.burnin, n.thin, DIC=TRUE)
attach.bugs(chemo2$BUGSoutput)
```

First, we "detach" all the objects obtained as output of the `jags` function that were previously attached to the R workspace. This can be easily done using the self-explanatory command `detach.bugs()`. Then we set the node rho to the postulated value of 1 and define the data list. In this case, the object `dataJags` contains the same elements as for the analysis of the EVPPI. The model file is also the same.

As for the `inits`, we now define the function in a slightly different way: this time we initialise all the random quantities, including SE and A, while previously we let JAGS deal with them. Since A depends on SE, we first simulate the latter outside the outputs list. Then we assign the simulated values to the output SE and use it to simulate the output A.

The rest of the R code should be familiar by now, and defines the number of iterations, burn-in and thinning before launching the function `jags` to store the MCMC results in the object `chemo2`, which is then attached to the R workspace. At this point, we can redefine the cost and effectiveness measures and rerun the health economic analysis by typing the following R commands.

```
e <- c <- matrix(NA,chemo$BUGSoutput$n.sims,2)
e <- N - SE
for (t in 1:2) {
    c[,t] <- c.drug[t]*(N-SE[,t]) + (c.amb+c.drug[t])*A[,t] +
            (c.hosp+c.drug[t])*H[,t]
}
m2 <- bcea(e=e,c=c,ref=2,interventions=treats,
            Kmax=50000,Ktable=25000)
```

The command `plot(m2)` produces Figure 3.9.

In order compute the model average, we first need to define the weights as functions of the DIC associated with each model being compared. We can do so by typing the following in R.

```
d <- w <- numeric()
d[1] <- chemo$BUGSoutput$DIC
d[2] <- chemo2$BUGSoutput$DIC
dmin <- min(d)
w <- exp(-.5*(d-dmin))/sum(exp(-.5*(d-dmin)))
```

First, we define the vectors d and w. Then we assign the DIC (which is stored in the element BUGSoutput$DIC of each model object) to the first and second elements of the vector d. We can use these values to compute the minimum DIC in the variable dmin and the weights by using (3.17).

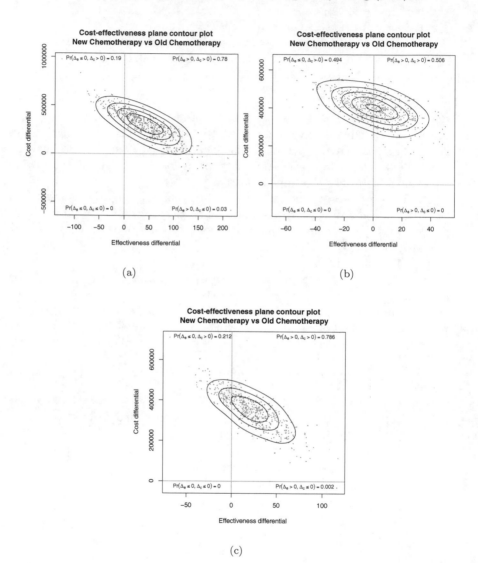

(a)   (b)

(c)

FIGURE 4.5
Contour plots for the joint distribution of (Δ_e, Δ_c): (a) original model; (b) model with ρ fixed to 1; and (c) model average.

Finally, we create new R variables SE, c.hosp, c.amb, A and H as the weighted average of the corresponding nodes for each of the two models being compared, where the weights are represented by the DIC-based values just computed.

```
SE <- w[1]*chemo$BUGSoutput$sims.list$SE +
      w[2]*chemo2$BUGSoutput$sims.list$SE
c.hosp <- w[1]*chemo$BUGSoutput$sims.list$c.hosp +
          w[2]*chemo2$BUGSoutput$sims.list$c.hosp
c.amb <- w[1]*chemo$BUGSoutput$sims.list$c.amb +
         w[2]*chemo2$BUGSoutput$sims.list$c.amb
A <- w[1]*chemo$BUGSoutput$sims.list$A +
     w[2]*chemo2$BUGSoutput$sims.list$A
H <- w[1]*chemo$BUGSoutput$sims.list$H +
     w[2]*chemo2$BUGSoutput$sims.list$H
```

These variables can be used to generate new measures of cost and effectiveness for the "average" model, which we use to rerun the health economic analysis, whose results we now save in the object m.avg.

```
e <- c <- matrix(NA,chemo$BUGSoutput$n.sims,2)
e <- N - SE
for (t in 1:2) {
    c[,t] <- c.drug[t]*(N-SE[,t]) + (c.amb+c.drug[t])*A[,t] +
             (c.hosp+c.drug[t])*H[,t]
}
m.avg <- bcea(e=e,c=c,ref=2,interventions=treats,
         Kmax=50000,Ktable=25000)
```

Figure 4.5 shows the contour plots for the joint distribution of (Δ_e, Δ_c) for the two models being compared in panels (a) and (b) and for the model average in panel (c). These are obtained using the function contour in the package bcea.

Since model $\mathcal{M}_1$ seems to be the most supported by the DIC-based procedure (cfr. the value of the weights in §3.6), the average is very similar to the original model. However, due to the impact of $\mathcal{M}_2$, there is a lower chance of $t = 1$ being cost-saving for the new drugs in the average model than in $\mathcal{M}_1$.

5

Health economic evaluation in practice

5.1 Introduction

In this final chapter we present some examples of health economic evaluation. In particular we focus on three "typical" cases; the first concerns the analysis of individual level data, specifically from a RCT, in which a sample of individuals is observed in terms of the relevant measures of cost and clinical outcome. The second example focusses on the process of evidence synthesis, a situation particularly relevant when individual data are not available. In these situations, the relevant random quantities can be estimated by the combination of the available evidence, e.g. coming from published studies, or expert opinions. Within the Bayesian framework, this is very much linked to the development of hierarchical models, which we briefly review before presenting the example. Finally, we consider the analysis of Markov models, an increasingly popular tool in health economic evaluation, which allow the simulation of a followup analysis on a "virtual" cohort of patients.

While the problems highlighted in each of the following sections can be considered as typical of the situations considered in applied health economics, they are far from representing an exhaustive set: in real applications, there are countless subtleties and nuisances that need to be addressed specifically. In particular in the Bayesian approach, this requires a careful specification of the model to be used, mainly in terms of the prior distributions, but also in terms of the possible correlation levels among the observed and unobserved random variables.

Nevertheless, we tackle some of the most relevant issues arising from the analysis of health economic data, trying to point out possible solutions and references where more detailed modelling strategies are presented. All the examples are worked out starting from the description of the problem, the specification of the Bayesian model, and then the code used to run the MCMC analysis and the post-processing necessary to derive the relevant health economic quantities used to produce the decision-making process.

5.2   Cost-effectiveness analysis alongside clinical trials

One of the most interesting characteristic of clinical trial data is the availability of suitable measures of effectiveness and costs observed as individual records. In other words, for each patient $i = 1, \ldots, n_t$ under intervention $t \in \mathcal{T}$, we have available a pair of observations (e_i, c_i).

In almost all circumstances, it is plausible to assume that the variables of effectiveness and cost are correlated, which implies an underlying bivariate distribution to model the outcomes. Assuming no correlation across interventions, the easiest way of formalising the problem is to consider for each strategy t a joint bivariate Normal distribution (van Hout et al., 1994)

$$(e, c \mid \boldsymbol{\mu}, \boldsymbol{\Sigma}) \sim \text{Normal}(\boldsymbol{\mu}, \boldsymbol{\Sigma}),$$

where $\boldsymbol{\mu} = (\mu_e, \mu_c)$ is the vector of population averages for the benefits and costs and

$$\boldsymbol{\Sigma} = \begin{pmatrix} \sigma_e^2 & \rho\sigma_e\sigma_c \\ \rho\sigma_e\sigma_c & \sigma_c^2 \end{pmatrix}$$

is the population covariance matrix. Here, σ_e^2 and σ_c^2 quantify the variability *within* the measures of benefit and cost, while ρ represents the level of correlation *between* them.

One possible way to simplify the modelling of individual level data is to consider a regression formulation, in which the joint distribution $p(e, c)$ is factorised in the product of a marginal and a conditional distribution, e.g. $p(e)p(c \mid e)$. In the simple case of the bivariate Normal model, this translates into a marginal distribution for the variable of effectiveness

$$e_i \sim \text{Normal}\left(\mu_e, \sigma_e^2\right) \tag{5.1}$$

and a conditional distribution for the costs

$$c_i \mid e_i \sim \text{Normal}\left(\mu_c + \frac{\sigma_c}{\sigma_e}\rho(e_i - \mu_e), \sigma_c^2(1 - \rho)\right). \tag{5.2}$$

While the use of Normal distribution for both cost and benefit is in many cases not reasonable, it is possible to generalise this model to a large set of parametric distributions, expressing the mean of the conditional distribution in terms of the parameters of the joint model, as in (5.2). Therefore this modelling strategy proves particularly helpful in dealing with individual data, e.g. from RCTs.

Thompson and Nixon (2005) apply this method to model the joint distribution for cost and benefit using two possible strategies. The first one consists of a Gamma marginal distribution for the cost and a Gamma conditional distribution for the measure of effectiveness. The second model considers a logNormal marginal distribution for the cost and a Normal conditional distribution for the benefit.

Willan et al. (2004) and Nixon and Thompson (2005) extend this framework to adjust for covariates. This is particularly relevant when individual data are available in non-experimental settings, where randomisation has not been performed and therefore there could be unbalance among the different treatment groups.

5.2.1 Example: RCT of acupuncture for chronic headache in primary care

We consider here a RCT conducted in the UK primary care setting to evaluate the cost-effectiveness of acupuncture in the management of chronic headache. The study is originally presented in Wonderling et al. (2004).

The trial recruited a total of 401 patients aged 18–65 who reported an average of at least two headaches per month, from general practices in England and Wales. The participants were randomly allocated to either usual care (which we indicate with $t = 0$), or in addition up to 12 acupuncture treatments over three months from appropriately trained physiotherapists (active intervention, $t = 1$).

The measure of effectiveness used in the study is the total QALYs gained. This was obtained using a specific algorithm based on SF-6D questionnaires (cfr. §1.4.3). Only 255 patients (119 in the control and 136 in the active treatment group) had valid data for the SF-6D questionnaire and thus the economic evaluation is performed on this sub-sample. Notice that because the time horizon considered is one year and the SF-6D utility measure is defined in the interval $[0; 1]$, the resulting QALYs for each individual are constrained in this interval.

The overall cost was calculated for each patient by adding up the following resources: *i)* non-prescription drugs and private health care visits (reported by the patients); *ii)* visits to practitioners of complementary or alternative medicine. The unit cost included overheads, capital and training, and the total cost was obtained by multiplying this by the contact time for each individual patient with the physiotherapist trained in acupuncture; and *iii)* drug prescriptions (obtained from the general practitioner database). The distribution of costs for the two groups is presented in Figure 1.2.

5.2.2 Model description

We use a formulation similar to (5.1) and (5.2). In this case, the assumption of normality is unrealistic for both the quantities of interest. In fact, the benefits are measured in terms of QALYs on a scale $[0; 1]$, while the costs are as usual defined on the positive axis. Thus, direct application of the bivariate Normal model is not correct.

However, we can apply suitable transformations to the raw data in order to re-scale the variables (e, c) on $(-\infty; \infty)$ and to induce symmetry, at least to a reasonably degree of approximation, so that normality is justified on the transformed scale.

For each strategy, we compute two new variables:

$$e^* = \text{logit}(e) = \log\left(\frac{e}{1-e}\right)$$

represents the QALYs on the logit scale, while

$$c^* = \log(c + \epsilon),$$

represents the costs on the log scale. Here, $\epsilon > 0$ is added to each original cost to avoid problems related to 4 patients who had originally incurred no cost at all (and therefore the log of their cost would be $-\infty$, leading to estimation inconsistencies). Notice that the analysis is possibly sensitive to the value of ϵ and therefore it will be necessary to study and report this aspect in the full economic evaluation. In the base-case, we assume $\epsilon = 1$.

For each strategy $t = (0, 1)$ we model the pair (e^*, c^*) using the following specification:

$$e_{it}^* \sim \text{Normal}\left(\mu_{et}, \sigma_{et}^2\right) \tag{5.3}$$
$$c_{it}^* \mid e_{it}^* \sim \text{Normal}\left(\phi_{it}, \psi_t^2\right),$$

where the conditional mean for the log cost is defined using the linear regression

$$\phi_{it} = \mu_{ct} + \beta_t \left(e_{it}^* - \mu_{et}\right). \tag{5.4}$$

In line with (5.2), the parameters

$$\beta_t = \frac{\sigma_{ct}}{\sigma_{et}}\rho$$

(with σ_{ct}^2 and ρ representing the marginal variance of the log costs and the correlation between logit QALYs and log costs, respectively) quantify the association between costs and benefits. Moreover, the conditional variance for the log cost $\psi_t^2 = \sigma_{ct}^2(1 - \rho^2)$ can be re-expressed in terms of the parameters β_t as

$$\psi_t^2 = \sigma_{ct}^2 - \sigma_{et}^2\beta_t^2. \tag{5.5}$$

To complete the Bayesian model, we need to include suitable priors for the parameters of interest. In this case, these are represented by the vectors $\boldsymbol{\theta}^t = (\mu_{et}, \sigma_{et}, \mu_{ct}, \sigma_{ct}, \beta_t)$ since, as appears clear from (5.4) and (5.5), the remaining parameters (ϕ_{it}, ψ_t^2) are in fact deterministic functions of $\boldsymbol{\theta}^t$.

We use independent minimally informative priors for the means

$$\mu_{et} \sim \text{Normal}(0, v) \quad \text{and} \quad \mu_{ct} \sim \text{Normal}(0, v),$$

with v a large constant value to express the prior variance, e.g. $v = 1\,000\,000$. In this case, since both μ_{et} and μ_{ct} represent the average on a Normal (transformed) scale, we can use a Normal prior with large variance to encode the lack of clear knowledge.

Similarly, we adopt relatively vague independent priors on the logarithm of the standard deviations

$$\log(\sigma_{et}) \sim \text{Uniform}(-5, 10) \quad \text{and} \quad \log(\sigma_{ct}) \sim \text{Uniform}(-5, 10)$$

and on the regression coefficient: $\beta_t \sim \text{Uniform}(-5, 5)$.

Again, notice that σ_{et} and σ_{ct} are standard deviations on a Normal scale and thus the prior range is very large. This allows us to encode weak information in these priors. Moreover, the parameters β_t effectively represent the regression coefficient in a regression model defined on a log-scale and including an intercept, cfr. (5.4). Thus, its value is unlikely to be greater than ± 5 and therefore the range assumed in the prior ensures that only minimal information is induced. As always, sensitivity to this choice should be checked in the absence of more substantial information about the plausible range of β_t.

5.2.3 JAGS implementation

The model, which we label as $\mathcal{M}_1$, is implemented in JAGS using the following code, where the quantities c0[i] and c1[i] represent respectively c_{i0}^* and c_{i1}^*. Similarly, e0[i] and e1[i] are used for e_{i0}^* and e_{i1}^*.

```
model {
# Controls
    for(i in 1:n[1]){
        c0[i] ~ dnorm(phi0[i],lambda[1])
        e0[i] ~ dnorm(mu.e[1],tau[1])
        phi0[i] <- mu.c[1]+beta[1]*(e0[i]-mu.e[1])
    }
# Treatments
    for(i in 1:n[2]){
        c1[i] ~ dnorm(phi1[i],lambda[2])
        e1[i] ~ dnorm(mu.e[2],tau[2])
        phi1[i] <- mu.c[2]+beta[2]*(e1[i]-mu.e[2])
    }

    for (t in 1:2) {
# Conditional precision and variance for costs
        lambda[t] <- 1/psi1[t]
        psi1[t] <- sigma2.c[t]-sigma2.e[t]*pow(beta[t],2)

# Marginal variance and standard deviation for costs
        sigma2.c[t] <- pow(sigma.c[t],2)
        sigma.c[t] <- exp(logsigma.c[t])

# Precision, variance and standard deviation for QALYs
        tau[t] <- pow(sigma.e[t],-2)
        sigma2.e[t] <- pow(sigma.e[t],2)
```

```
              sigma.e[t] <- exp(logsigma.e[t])

# Prior distributions
              mu.c[t] ~ dnorm(0, 1.0E-6)        # mean costs (log scale)
              logsigma.c[t] ~ dunif(-5,10)      # log st. dev. for costs
              mu.e[t] ~ dnorm(0, 1.0E-6)        # mean QALY (logit scale)
              logsigma.e[t] ~ dunif(-5,10)      # log st. dev. for QALYs
              beta[t] ~ dunif(-5, 5)            # regression between (e,c)
       }
}
```

Notice that we need to define the nodes `lambda[t]` to model the precision of the conditional distributions for c_{it}^*. Obviously, its value is set to the reciprocal of the conditional variance.

We save the code in the file `acupt.txt` and run the model in JAGS using the following code.

```
library(R2jags)
dataJags <- list("n","c0","c1","e0","e1")
filein <- "acuptRCT.txt"
params <- c("mu.c","mu.e","beta","sigma.e","sigma.c")
inits <- function(){
    list(
        mu.c=rnorm(2,0,1),mu.e=rnorm(2,0,1),
        beta=runif(2,-0.5,0.5),logsigma.c=runif(2,0,1),
        logsigma.e=runif(2,0,1)
    )
}

n.iter <- 10000
n.burnin <- 5000
n.thin <- floor((n.iter-n.burnin)/500)
acupt <- jags(data=dataJags,inits,params,filein,
    n.chains=2,n.iter,n.burnin,n.thin,DIC=TRUE)
print(acupt,digits=3,intervals=c(0.025, 0.975))
attach.bugs(acupt$BUGSoutput)
```

This produces the summary table with the statistics for all the parameters monitored.

```
Inference for Bugs model at "acuptRCT.txt", fit using jags,
 2 chains, each with 10000 iterations (first 5000 discarded),
 n.thin = 10, n.sims = 1000 iterations saved
              mu.vect sd.vect     2.5%     97.5% Rhat n.eff
beta[1]        -0.311   0.202   -0.697    0.094 1.001  1000
beta[2]        -0.168   0.091   -0.347    0.009 1.000  1000
mu.c[1]         4.546   0.138    4.283    4.807 1.006   240
mu.c[2]         5.752   0.068    5.629    5.885 1.001  1000
mu.e[1]         0.971   0.061    0.852    1.086 1.000  1000
mu.e[2]         1.095   0.066    0.966    1.224 1.001  1000
```

```
sigma.c[1]    1.475    0.099    1.299    1.684 1.005     310
sigma.c[2]    0.814    0.052    0.722    0.923 1.001    1000
sigma.e[1]    0.644    0.044    0.569    0.737 1.001    1000
sigma.e[2]    0.756    0.045    0.673    0.851 1.002    1000
deviance   1292.077    4.727 1285.271 1302.588 1.001    1000

For each parameter, n.eff is a crude measure of effective sample size,
and Rhat is the potential scale reduction factor
(at convergence, Rhat=1).

DIC info (using the rule, pD = var(deviance)/2)
pD = 11.2 and DIC = 1303.3
DIC is an estimate of expected predictive error
(lower deviance is better).
```

Convergence is reasonably reached as all the monitored parameters show a value for the $\hat{R}$ statistic well below the threshold of 1.1. The command attach.bugs(acupt$BUGSoutput) finally makes the output of the model available to R.

5.2.4 Cost-effectiveness analysis

The cost-effectiveness analysis relies on the population averages for the measure of cost and clinical benefit, both computed on the natural scale. Thus, it is necessary to transform the means obtained from the model (which are defined on the logit and log scale for QALYs and costs, respectively) back to the natural scale.

Because the transformation used to create (e^*, c^*) is non linear, we need to be careful in computing the averages on the correct scale. Using the mathematical properties of the logNormal distribution, it is straightforward to compute the mean cost by applying the inverse transformation

$$m_{ct} = \exp\left(\mu_{ct} + \frac{1}{2}\sigma_{ct}^2\right). \tag{5.6}$$

Notice that because there are n_{sims} simulations from the posterior distribution of $(\mu_{ct}, \sigma_{ct}^2)$, equation (5.6) effectively produces a sample from the induced posterior distribution of m_{ct}.

The computation is more complex for the QALYs, since there is no analytical form in which we can define the mean on the natural scale as a function of the parameters on the logit scale. However, it is possible to use the results from the model to obtain the required estimation by means of Monte Carlo integration.

First, we define the number of Monte Carlo simulations, n_{MC}; of course, as suggested in Table 2.4, the larger this value, the better the resulting approximation to the required quantity. Then, for each value $s = 1, \ldots, n_{\text{sim}}$ simulated from the posterior distribution of $(\mu_{et}, \sigma_{et}^2)$, we compute a vector of n_{MC} draws from the predictive distribution $\mathbf{e}_{st}^{*pred} = (e_{1st}^{*pred}, \ldots, e_{n_{MC}st}^{*pred})$.

Next, we can transform the predictive values from the logit to the natural scale by applying the inverse logit function

$$\mathbf{e}_{st}^{pred} = \frac{\exp\left(\mathbf{e}_{st}^{*pred}\right)}{1 + \exp\left(\mathbf{e}_{st}^{*pred}\right)}.$$

Similarly to what we did for the costs, we have now effectively generated a sample of $(n_{sims} \times n_{MC})$ simulations for the QALYs on the natural scale. Finally, we can estimate the posterior distribution of the mean on the natural scale by computing for each $s = 1, \ldots, n_{sims}$ the sample mean over the n_{MC} simulations

$$m_{et} = \left(\frac{1}{n_{MC}} \sum_{l=1}^{n_{MC}} e_{l1t}^{pred}, \ldots, \frac{1}{n_{MC}} \sum_{l=1}^{n_{MC}} e_{ln_{sim}t}^{pred}\right).$$

The above computations can be done in R using the following syntax.

```
#1. Defines the mean costs and QALYs on the natural scale
m.c <- m.e <- matrix(NA,acupt$BUGSoutput$n.sims,2)


#2. Estimate the mean cost on the natural scale
for (t in 1:2) {
    m.c[,t] <- exp(mu.c[,t]+0.5*(sigma.c[,t])^2)
}


#3. Estimate the mean QALYs on the natural scale
estar.pred <- e.pred <- array(NA,c(n.MC,n.sims,2))
for (t in 1:2) {
    for (s in 1:n.sims) {
        estar.pred[,s,t] <- rnorm(n.MC,mu.e[s,t],sigma.e[s,t])
        e.pred[,s,t] <- exp(estar.pred[,s,t]) /
                            (1+exp(estar.pred[,s,t]))
    }
    m.e[,t] <- apply(e.pred[,,t],2,mean)
}
```

First, the population average for the costs is easily calculated by directly coding equation (5.6). Then, we compute the predictive values on the logit and natural scale and finally we use the function apply to produce the estimation of the population average for the QALYs. Notice that the quantities estar.pred are computed by simulating n.MC values from a Normal distribution with mean and standard deviation equal to the s-th value of the vector of simulations from the posterior distribution of μ_{et} and of σ_{et}, respectively.

For convenience, we next build the matrices e <- cbind(m.e[,1],m.e[,2]) and c <- cbind(m.c[,1],m.c[,2]), as well as the vector of labels ints <- c("Treatment as usual","Acupuncture") for the two interventions and finally launch the function bcea to perform the cost-effectiveness analysis.

```
he <- bcea(e,c,ref=2,interventions=ints)
```

Figure 5.1 shows the results in terms of the cost-effectiveness plane and the EIB, CEAC and EVPI as functions of the willingness to pay parameter (set in the interval £[0; 50 000]).

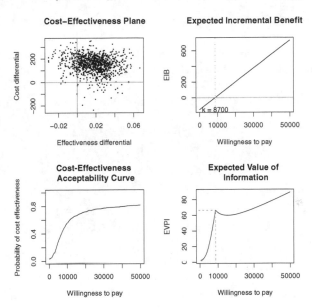

FIGURE 5.1
Summary of the health economic evaluation for the acupuncture model.

As appears clear, already for relatively low values of the willingness-to-pay threshold ($k \geq 8\,700$), $t = 1$ is the most cost-effective intervention, producing a likely increase in the overall cost, which is compensated by a likely increase in the clinical benefits, as suggested by the analysis of the cost-effectiveness plane.

The analysis of the CEAC shows that the probability of cost-effectiveness is relatively high and over 0.8 in the limit (i.e. for $k \geq 30\,000$). Similarly, the EVPI is quite low — at the point of maximum uncertainty it is just above £80 per patient.

5.2.5 Alternative specifications of the model

As suggested earlier, other possible distributions can be used to model the costs and benefits. In particular, the results might be quite sensitive to the assumed distribution for the costs and therefore it is useful to check this aspect of the modelling.

Following Thompson and Nixon (2005), we tested two different model specifications in which, while the assumed distribution for the QALYs is unchanged, the costs are modelled using a Gamma and a logNormal distribution, respectively.

Normal/Gamma model on the logit/natural scale

Since we are now using a Gamma distribution, defined in the interval $(0; +\infty)$, the costs can theoretically be modelled directly with no need to apply transformations to fit the support of the assumed distribution. However, because of the patients with observed 0 costs, we still need to add a small value ϵ to c, in order to run the Gamma model. Thus, we define the new variable $c^* = c + \epsilon$.

The model for the QALYs is the same as in (5.3), while we assume

$$
\begin{aligned}
c_{it}^* \mid e_{it}^* \;\sim\;& \text{Gamma}\,(\eta_t, \lambda_{it}) \\
=\;& \lambda_{it}^{\eta_t} \frac{1}{\Gamma(\eta_t)} c_{it}^{*(\eta_t - 1)} e^{-\lambda_{it} c_{it}^*}.
\end{aligned}
$$

In line with BUGS/WinBUGS and JAGS requirements, we characterise the Gamma distribution in terms of a *shape* parameter η_t and a *rate* λ_{it}. By the mathematical properties of the Gamma density, this is defined as

$$
\lambda_{it} = \frac{\eta_t}{\phi_{it}},
$$

where ϕ_{it} is the mean of the cost conditional distribution, which we model as in (5.4).

Suitable priors need to be defined on the parameters of this model which we indicate as $\boldsymbol{\theta}^t = (\eta_t, \mu_{ct}, \mu_{et}, \sigma_{et}, \beta_t)$; the additional parameters λ_{it} and ϕ_{it} are defined as deterministic functions of $\boldsymbol{\theta}^t$ and therefore do not require a prior distribution.

We use the same prior specifications as in §5.2.2 for μ_{et}, σ_{et} and β_t. Moreover, since by definition of the Gamma density the shape parameters η_t need to have strictly positive values, in order to imply minimal information in the prior we use a Uniform distribution defined in a large enough, positive interval. In the base-case we select $[0, 100]$, but sensitivity analysis should be performed to check that this choice really generates a weak prior distribution.

Finally, we need to define a prior distribution on μ_{ct}, the population mean cost; this is a positive quantity and thus a Uniform distribution on a relatively large and positive range can be considered as a reasonable minimally informative prior. In this case we choose the interval $[0; 2000]$, using some prior knowledge about the expected cost of patients with chronic headache.

We label this model $\mathcal{M}_2$ and its JAGS implementation is shown below.

```
model {
# Controls
    for(i in 1:n[1]){
        c0[i] ~ dgamma(eta[1],lambda0[i])
        lambda0[i] <- eta[1] / phi0[i]
```

```
        e0[i] ~ dnorm(mu.e[1],tau[1])
        phi0[i] <- mu.c[1]+beta[1]*(e0[i]-mu.e[1])
    }
# Treatments
    for(i in 1:n[2]){
        c1[i] ~ dgamma(eta[2],lambda1[i])
        lambda1[i] <- eta[2] / phi1[i]
        e1[i] ~ dnorm(mu.e[2],tau[2])
        phi1[i] <- mu.c[2]+beta[2]*(e1[i]-mu.e[2])
    }

    for (t in 1:2) {
        tau[t] <- pow(sigma.e[t],-2)      # precision for QALYs
        sigma2.e[t] <- pow(sigma.e[t],2)  # variance for QALYs
        sigma.e[t] <- exp(logsigma.e[t])  # st.dev. for QALYs

# Prior distributions
        eta[t] ~ dunif(0,100)         # shape parameter of Gamma dist.
        mu.c[t] ~ dunif(0,2000)       # mean cost (normal scale)
        mu.e[t] ~ dnorm(0, 1.0E-6)    # mean QALY (logit scale)
        logsigma.e[t] ~ dunif(-5,10)  # log-st.dev. for QALYs
        beta[t] ~ dunif(-5,5)         # regression between (e,c)
    }

}
```

Normal/logNormal model on the logit/natural scale

In this final model specification we reverse the modelling strategy and factorise the joint distribution $p(e, c)$ as the product $p(c)p(e \mid c)$; in other words, we first define a marginal distribution for the costs and then a conditional distribution for the QALYs, given the observed value of the costs.

Since the logNormal model can be used for positive and skewed variables, we can again model the costs directly (with the usual addition of the quantity ϵ to correct for observed zeros), while we keep the logit-Normal formulation for the QALYs.

The pair (e^*, c^*) is then modelled according to the following specification. The marginal distribution for the costs is

$$
\begin{aligned}
c_{it}^* &\sim \text{logNormal}(\nu_{it}, \sigma_{ct}^2) \\
&= \frac{1}{c_{it}^* \sqrt{2\pi\sigma_{ct}^2}} \exp\left(-\frac{[\log(c_{it}^*) - \nu_{it}]^2}{2\sigma_{ct}^2}\right),
\end{aligned}
$$

where the parameters ν_{it} and σ_{ct}^2 represent the mean and the variance on the log scale. Using the same argument in (5.6), it is possible to express the mean on the log scale as a function of the population mean μ_{ct} as

$$
\nu_{it} = \log(\mu_{ct}) - \frac{1}{2}\sigma_{ct}^2.
$$

As for the logit-QALYs, we use the following conditional distribution

$$
e_{it}^* \mid c_{it} \sim \text{Normal}(\phi_{it}, \sigma_{et}^2),
$$

where the conditional mean is modelled through the regression

$$\phi_{it} = \mu_{et} + \beta_t(c_{it} - \mu_{ct}).$$

Notice here that we do not necessarily need to include in the model the variances (or standard deviations) for both QALYs and costs on the natural scale. In fact, the model just described considers these parameters on the logit and log scale, respectively. However, using suitable back transformations, it would be possible to include in the MCMC simulation two additional nodes to monitor the variances on the natural scale.

In this model, the parameters to be given a prior distribution are $\theta^t = (\mu_{et}, \sigma_{et}, \mu_{ct}, \sigma_{ct}, \beta_t)$, while (ϕ_t, ν_t) are defined deterministically. Effectively all prior distributions are the same as in §5.2.2, except for μ_{ct}. In fact, now this parameter is the mean of a variable associated with a logNormal distribution and as such it has to be confined to take values on the positive line. Similarly to the Gamma case, a reasonable minimally informative prior is represented by a Uniform distribution in a large enough range (and for the sake of simplicity, we select again the interval $[0; 2000]$).

The JAGS code to represent this model (which we label as $\mathcal{M}_3$) is shown below.

```
model {
# Controls
    for(i in 1:n[1]){
        c0[i] ~ dlnorm(nu0[i],tau.c[1])
        e0[i] ~ dnorm(phi0[i],tau.e[1])
        phi0[i] <- mu.e[1]+beta[1]*(c0[i]-mu.c[1])
        nu0[i] <- log(mu.c[1])-0.5*sigma2.c[1]
    }

# Treatments
    for(i in 1:n[2]){
        c1[i] ~ dlnorm(nu1[i],tau.c[2])
        e1[i] ~ dnorm(phi1[i],tau.e[2])
        phi1[i] <- mu.e[2]+beta[2]*(c1[i]-mu.c[2])
        nu1[i] <- log(mu.c[2])-0.5*sigma2.c[2]
    }

    for (t in 1:2) {
        tau.c[t] <- pow(sigma.c[t],-2)    # precision for log costs
        sigma2.c[t] <- pow(sigma.c[t],2)  # variance for log costs
        sigma.c[t] <- exp(logsigma.c[t])  # st.dev. for log costs

        tau.e[t] <- pow(sigma.e[t],-2)    # precision for QALYs
        sigma2.e[t] <- pow(sigma.e[t],2)  # variance for QALYs
        sigma.e[t] <- exp(logsigma.e[t])  # st.dev. for QALYs

# Prior distributions
        mu.c[t] ~ dunif(low,upp)          # mean costs (natural scale)
        logsigma.c[t] ~ dunif(-5,10)      # log-st.dev. for costs
        mu.e[t] ~ dnorm(0, 1.0E-6)        # mean QALY (logit scale)
        logsigma.e[t] ~ dunif(-5,10)      # log-st.dev. for QALYs
        beta[t] ~ dunif(-5, 5)            # regression between (e,c)
```

```
    }
}
```

Cost-effectiveness analysis

In both the alternative models, the measure of effectiveness obtained by the implementation of the Bayesian model needs to be back transformed into the natural scale (since it was originally defined on the logit scale), while the costs are already on the correct dimension.

Thus, in both cases, once the MCMC simulations are made available to the R workspace we can type the following code

```
for (t in 1:2) {
    m.c[,t] <- mu.c[,t]
}
estar.pred <- e.pred <- array(NA,c(n.MC,n.sims,2))
for (t in 1:2) {
    for (s in 1:n.sims) {
        estar.pred[,s,t] <- rnorm(n.MC,mu.e[s,t],sigma.e[s,t])
        e.pred[,s,t] <- exp(estar.pred[,s,t]) /
                        (1+exp(estar.pred[,s,t]))
    }
    m.e[,t] <- apply(e.pred[,,t],2,mean)
}

e <- cbind(m.e[,1],m.e[,2])
c <- cbind(m.c[,1],m.c[,2])
```

and then run the function bcea using the quantities e and c as input to perform the cost-effectiveness analysis.

Table 5.1 shows a comparison of the summary statistics for the posterior distributions of the population averages of costs and benefits for the three models being investigated.

Models $\mathcal{M}_1$ and $\mathcal{M}_3$ give very similar results. This is plausible, since they have effectively the same specification, in that they both use a Normal model for the log costs. Model $\mathcal{M}_2$, however, provides slightly different results for the costs.

As discussed in §3.6, it is generally useful to perform PSA to the structural assumptions, e.g. producing a model average accounting for the different results obtained by the three different structures analysed. In this particular case, as shown in Figure 5.2, despite the differences highlighted in Table 5.1, the impact on the decision process does not seem to be very significant.

Models $\mathcal{M}_1$ and $\mathcal{M}_3$ effectively produce the same break-even points. For larger values of the break-even point, the differences between $\mathcal{M}_2$ and $\mathcal{M}_3$ tend to become smaller in terms of the EIB. With respect to the EVPI, the range of values obtained comparing the different models is all in all not too relevant. Overall, the general interpretation of the results is that $t = 1$ is a

TABLE 5.1

Summary statistics from the posterior distributions of the population average for cost and QALYs, computed starting from the simulations of the model parameters. Models $\mathcal{M}_1$ and $\mathcal{M}_3$ produce nearly identical results, while model $\mathcal{M}_2$ estimates lower costs for both interventions.

Variable	Mean	SD	95% Credible interval	
$\mathcal{M}_1$: Normal/Normal model on logit/log scale				
m_{c0}	286.67	61.02	196.66	438.72
m_{c1}	441.22	35.89	380.20	516.28
m_{e0}	0.724	0.012	0.700	0.748
m_{e1}	0.749	0.012	0.725	0.772
$\mathcal{M}_2$: Normal/Gamma model on logit/natural scale				
m_{c0}	223.38	25.46	178.77	279.81
m_{c1}	406.06	24.17	361.81	454.43
m_{e0}	0.725	0.011	0.702	0.748
m_{e1}	0.750	0.012	0.726	0.773
$\mathcal{M}_3$: Normal/logNormal model on logit/natural scale				
m_{c0}	294.90	62.14	202.58	442.51
m_{c1}	441.71	36.04	377.17	518.92
m_{e0}	0.721	0.012	0.697	0.744
m_{e1}	0.746	0.013	0.721	0.770

cost-effective intervention and that the uncertainty underlying this judgement is relatively limited.   □

As suggested earlier, the inclusion of the constant ϵ to avoid estimation problems due to patients with observed zero-costs can be problematic, since the results may strongly depend on the chosen value. More appropriately, it is possible to use specific strategies to model data including null costs, e.g. *hurdle* models (see for example Ntzoufras, 2009 for some examples of hurdle models developed in a Bayesian setting).

These generally consist of two parts that are connected to form a full Bayesian model; extensive treatment of this topic in the health economics literature is given in Cooper et al. (2003) and Cooper et al. (2007).

To simplify the notation, we define the available data as $\mathcal{D} = (\mathcal{D}_{pos} \cup \mathcal{D}_{null})$ where $\mathcal{D}_{pos}$ represents the data on the n_{pos} subjects with positive costs and $\mathcal{D}_{null}$ includes the data for the $(n - n_{pos})$ subjects with zero costs. The first model is a logistic regression to predict which individuals experience positive costs, for instance based on some relevant covariates.

For each of the $i = 1, \ldots, n$ subjects in the sample, we define an indicator variable d_i taking value 1 if the observed cost is positive and 0 otherwise. This

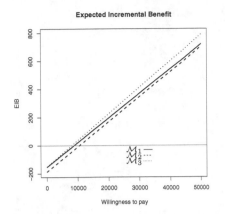
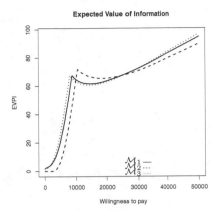

FIGURE 5.2
Comparison of the impact of different structural assumptions on the decision process, represented by the EIB and the EVPI. For models $\mathcal{M}_1$ and $\mathcal{M}_3$ the break-even point is nearly identical, while it is slightly larger for model $\mathcal{M}_2$.

is modelled as

$$d_i \sim \text{Bernoulli}(\pi_i)$$

$$\text{logit}(\pi_i) = \alpha_0 + \sum_{j=1}^{J} \alpha_j x_{ij},$$

where π_i is the individual probability of producing positive costs and $\mathbf{x}_i = (x_{i1}, \dots, x_{iJ})$ is a set of J relevant covariates (e.g. individual age, sex, comorbidities, etc.).

The second part models the distribution of costs for the subjects in $\mathcal{D}_{pos}$ only. For example, for each of the $i = 1, \dots, n_{pos}$ subjects with positive costs, we could define

$$c_i \mid c_i > 0 \sim \text{logNormal}(\mu_i, \sigma^2)$$

$$\mu_i = \beta_0 + \sum_{l=1}^{L} \beta_l z_{il},$$

where now μ_i is the average cost (in this case on the log scale) and $\mathbf{z}_i = (z_{i1}, \dots, z_{iL})$ is a set of L relevant covariates (which may include some of the variables in $\mathbf{x}_i$). Of course, alternative specifications can be used for the costs (e.g. Gamma or other continuous, skewed distributions).

If data on $\mathbf{z}_i$ are available for the $(n - n_{pos})$ subjects with null costs, it is possible to use the posterior distribution of $\beta = (\beta_0, \ldots, \beta_L)$, which is derived from the data in $\mathcal{D}_{pos}$, to compute the predictive distribution

$$\mu_i^* = \beta_0 + \sum_{l=1}^{L} \beta_l z_{il}^*,$$

where z_{il}^* is the value of the l−th covariate measured on the i−th individual in $\mathcal{D}_{null}$.

This can in turn be used to estimate the cost for the subjects in $\mathcal{D}_{null}$ in terms of a mixture of the two components as

$$c_i^* = \pi_i \times \exp\left(\mu_i^* + \frac{\sigma^2}{2}\right) + (1 - \pi_i) \times 0. \tag{5.7}$$

Of course, if different specifications are used for the cost distribution, it is necessary to modify (5.7) to rescale the costs on the natural scale.

In addition, the different models can be formally assessed in terms of their predictive performance using tools such as *posterior predictive checks* (Gelman et al., 2004). These entail the comparison of (some aspects of) the model to the data actually observed. For example, we could obtain a sample from the predictive distribution of the variables (e^*, c^*), suitably rescale its components and compare them to the actually observed data (e, c) in order to assess model fitting.

As highlighted earlier, in the health economics case, this aspect cannot be divorced from the overall impact on the resulting decision-making process: two competing models may give results that are substantially different in terms of the estimation of the relevant parameters and perhaps of prediction; nevertheless, the actual impact on the health economic problem may not be too high, with one intervention clearly proving cost-effective without substantial uncertainty, irrespective of the model chosen.

5.3   Evidence synthesis and hierarchical models

As suggested by Spiegelhalter et al. (2004), it is unlikely that policies are informed by a single relevant study. Tools such as "meta-analysis" are commonly used in the medical statistics arena to summarise the available evidence with respect to a particular intervention.

The more general concept of *evidence synthesis*, originally developed by Eddy et al. (1990), is particularly relevant in the health economic evaluation setting (Ades and Sutton, 2006; Ades et al., 2006). The basic idea is to construct suitable models that allow studies of possibly different designs (e.g. RCT vs observational studies) to be pooled in order to estimate quantities of interest. These may include parameters relevant to a decision-analytic model that can be used to construct the measures of cost and effectiveness needed to perform an economic analysis. Thus, in a sense, meta-analyses can be considered as a special case of the more general tool provided by evidence synthesis.

When considering the possibility of synthesising several studies or evidence sources, there are a few possible models that can be used. The simplest is to assume that the observed data (e.g. in the form of summary statistics presented in published papers) are independent conditionally on a common parameter θ, as in Figure 5.3.

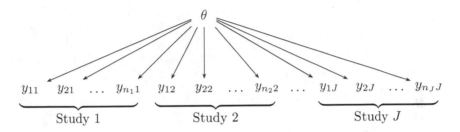

FIGURE 5.3
Graphical representation of the "complete pooling" analysis. All data *points* are considered to be independent and modelled assuming a unique data generating process, indexed by a common parameter θ.

In this situation, often referred to as *complete pooling*, the estimation is performed by combining all the data points, which generally leads to bias, when the observations are in fact correlated (e.g. by effect of some study-specific characteristics that may differ across the sources of evidence). In particular, the standard errors of the parameters tend to be underestimated, leading to overstatement of statistical significance.

A different specification considers the case where each data cluster (e.g. study) is assumed to have a fundamentally different nature, so that it is possible to model the values of each θ_j, i.e. the parameters of interest, as independent of each other. This situation is often referred to as *no pooling* (Figure 5.4).

Obviously, this modelling strategy might not be ideal either. In fact, while the correlation within each single study is accounted for by the use of the group-specific parameter θ_j, there is no means of using evidence from one group to inform the others, since we are effectively performing several separate analyses. This is not correct if there is reason to believe that the whole dataset is made by observations that share some common features (e.g. studies estimating some common parameter).

Hierarchical (or *multi-level*) models can be considered as a compromise between the two more extreme options of no- and complete-pooling. In this case, the J cluster-specific parameters are considered as exchangeable, i.e. as realisations of a common probability distribution (Figure 5.5).

By means of hierarchical modelling both possible levels of correlations

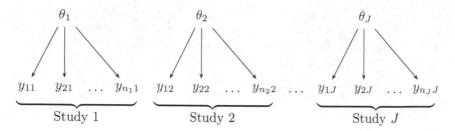

FIGURE 5.4
Graphical representation of the "no pooling" analysis. All data *clusters* are considered to be independent and modelled assuming a unique data generating process, indexed by a common parameter θ_j. These are in turn independent of each other and the information derived from one cluster bears no relevance to the others.

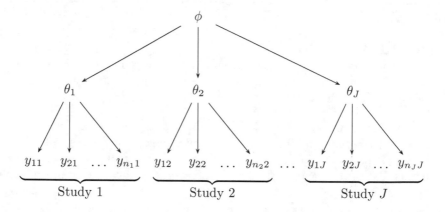

FIGURE 5.5
Graphical representation of the hierarchical analysis. Correlation within each data cluster is accounted for by the group-specific parameters θ_j. These are in turn considered to be exchangeable and characterised by a common hyper-parameter ϕ which allows the exchange of information from one group to the others.

(within and between clusters) are taken into account. The process of relating the different clusters in the hierarchical structure is sometimes referred to as "borrowing strength": it is still possible to learn about clusters made by only a few observations by obtaining some indirect evidence from the other (possibly larger) subgroups.

This feature is particularly relevant in the case of "indirect comparisons," where no head-to-head comparison between two interventions is available, but inference can be made using studies testing each of them against a common comparator (e.g. placebo, or treatment as usual).

In addition, both group-specific and overall parameters are estimated simulataneously in a hierarchical model. This can again represent an interesting feature, because both can be the main object of the analysis.

Bayesian modelling is particularly effective to represent multi-level data structures by exploiting exchangeability assumptions in the data. In the evidence synthesis setting, we typically assume the existence of J study, each reporting data on n_j units on which an outcome y_{ij} is observed. For example, this can be represented by the number of subjects presenting a characteristic of interest, or a suitable summary such as the median time to an event, or the mean value for some relevant measurement.

Each group is characterised by a parameter θ_j describing the variability within that study. In turns, the parameters in $\boldsymbol{\theta} = (\theta_1, \ldots, \theta_J)$ are modelled as draws from a probability distribution characterised by a vector of hyper-parameters ϕ. Thus, we encode the underlying assumptions of exchangeability: *i*) within each of the J groups, for the observed units; and *ii*) among the parameters in $\boldsymbol{\theta}$.

In general terms, a hierarchical structure is represented by first modelling the observed data $y_{ij} \sim p(y_{ij} \mid \theta_j)$ conditionally on the parameters θ_j. For example, this could be a Binomial distribution in the case where the data represent the observed number of patients with a given outcome, or a Normal distribution for continuous measurements.

Then (some function of) the parameters is associated with a probability distribution encoding the assumption of exchangeability. The easiest formulation is

$$g(\theta_j) \sim \text{Normal}(\mu_\theta, \sigma_\theta^2),$$

where for instance $g(\cdot)$ is the identity function for Normally distributed data, or the logit function for binary data, and $\phi = (\mu_\theta, \sigma_\theta^2)$ represents the vector of hyper-parameters identifying the common effect for all the studies (which is sometimes referred to as "pooled effect").

Finally, the model is completed by assigning a suitable probability distribution to ϕ, e.g. $\mu_\theta \sim \text{Normal}(0, v)$ and $\sigma_\theta \sim \text{Uniform}(0, h)$, for some fixed values v and h.

A popular terminology highlights the fact that the terms θ_js have a common distribution by referring to them as "*random effects*," in contrast to situations where the parameters are modelled independently, e.g. $g(\theta_j) \sim \text{Normal}(m, v)$ for some constant values m and v — and thus given the name of "*fixed effects*."

As suggested by Gelman and Hill (2007), within the Bayesian framework this is rather confusing. In fact, all parameters are given a probability distribution and thus they are all random quantities. It is the nature of the distribution (independent vs exchangeable) that makes a difference and therefore we prefer to indicate random or fixed effects as "*structured*" or "*unstructured*" effects, respectively.

The Bayesian procedure in evidence synthesis guarantees a better characterisation of the underlying variability in the structured parameters, which leads to better precision, e.g. estimations that tend to be unbiased and well calibrated, especially for non-Gaussian data (Browne and Draper, 2006). This is essentially due to the fact that the full uncertainty about the higher level parameters is reflected in the precision of the estimation, while in general non-Bayesian methods such as iterative generalised least squares (IGLS) or restricted maximum likelihood (REML) produce artificially narrow confidence intervals for the parameters of interest.

A further advantage of the Bayesian approach is the possibility of estimating functions of parameters in a relatively straightforward way. For example, by using an MCMC approach, it is sufficient to monitor some "fundamental" parameters θ and then define the parameter of actual interest ϕ using a suitable deterministic relationship $\phi = f(\theta)$. Uncertainty on ϕ is automatically accounted for. This aspect is discussed also in §5.4.6.

5.3.1   Example: Neuraminidase inhibitors to reduce influenza in healthy adults

Cooper et al. (2004) describe a model developed to quantify the cost-effectiveness of prophylactic use of neuraminidase inhibitors (NIs) to reduce the incidence of influenza A and B in healthy adults in the UK. NIs have been investigated and the evidence seems to suggest a reduction in the incidence of influenza during epidemic periods.

The model can be described by the simple graph in Figure 5.6. The possible interventions are $t = 0$, i.e. the status quo, where NIs are not used and $t = 1$, in which they are available. In either case, every single individual in the reference population can either have influenza (which happens with a probability p_t, varying in the two scenarios), or not, which of course has a probability of $1 - p_t$.

The model includes several cost components: first, the cost of acquisition of the NIs, which in the original analysis is assumed to be £2.40 per daily dose, bringing the total cost of a six weeks prophylactic course to £118.44, including the VAT (set at 17.5% as in the original paper). This is added to the cost of £19 for a GP consultation in which NIs are prescribed. Second, the cost of the treatment of a case of influenza is modelled using a Normal distribution with mean $\mu_{\text{inf}} = £16.78$ and standard deviation $\sigma_{\text{inf}} = £2.34$; these values are estimated using the published literature.

Clinical effectiveness is measured in terms of the length of time required to alleviate the symptoms of influenza, which we indicate as l. Summary statistics were computed on a set of observed data, which brought mean and standard deviation values on the natural scale of 8.2 days and $\sqrt{2}$ days, respectively. To account for the nature of this variable, l is given a logNormal distribution of mean μ_l and standard deviation σ_l, suitably defined to encode this prior knowledge.

Existing evidence in the form of published results is combined to estimate two remaining fundamental parameters in the model. First, a set of $H = 9$

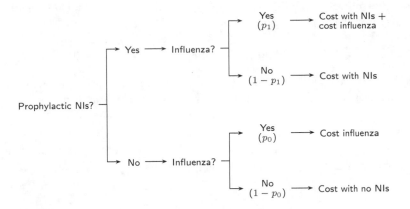

FIGURE 5.6
The model for the prophylactic use of NIs in influenza. For each clinical scenario, the cost is determined by the use of the relevant resources. The probability of the outcome (influenza) varies with the intervention.

studies is considered to evaluate the incidence of influenza in healthy adults, under the status quo. Then, the actual effectiveness of NIs in reducing the incidence of influenza (against no treatment) is evaluated by establishing a model to combine the results of $S = 6$ studies.

5.3.2 Model description

The model is made by several modules, each accounting for a different aspect. First we build the module to estimate the incidence of influenza. For each available study $h = 1, \ldots, H$, we observe results in the form of the number of patients who actually get influenza (x_h) out of a total number of patients observed, m_h. We model these using a Binomial specification

$$x_h \sim \text{Binomial}(\beta_h, m_h).$$

Here, β_h represents the population probability of influenza infection estimated from study h. In order to account for the correlation in the different studies, we assume a common Normal distribution on the logit scale

$$\text{logit}(\beta_h) = \gamma_h \sim \text{Normal}(\mu_\gamma, \sigma_\gamma^2)$$

(for simplicity in the notation we indicate this as a new variable γ_h). The parameter μ_γ represents the pooled mean probability of infection on the logit scale and thus we can rescale it to estimate

$$p_0 = \frac{\exp(\mu_\gamma)}{1 + \exp(\mu_\gamma)}.$$

The specification of this module is completed by including minimally informative prior distributions

$$\mu_\gamma \sim \text{Normal}(0, v) \qquad \text{and} \qquad \sigma_\gamma \sim \text{Uniform}(0, 10),$$

with $v = 1\,000\,000$ to encode the assumption of large prior variance.

The second module consists of the evidence synthesis used to estimate the comparative effectiveness of prophylactic treatment with NI (versus the status quo). For each study $s = 1, \ldots, S$ and for each treatment group we have available data on $r_s^{(t)}$, the number of patients who get infected out of the total number of patients $n_s^{(t)}$, which we again model using a Binomial specification

$$r_s^{(t)} \sim \text{Binomial}\left(\pi_s^{(t)}, n_s^{(t)}\right).$$

The parameters $\pi_s^{(t)}$ indicate the study- and treatment-specific chance of contracting influenza. Using again a logit specification, we model these as

$$\text{logit}(\pi_s^{(0)}) = \alpha_s \sim \text{Normal}(0, 10)$$
$$\text{logit}(\pi_s^{(1)}) = \alpha_s + \delta_s$$
$$\delta_s \sim \text{Normal}(\mu_\delta, \sigma_\delta^2).$$

The parameters α_s represent the baseline probability of influenza for the control group in study s; these are modelled as unstructured effects using a prior specification that assumes a fixed variance. Recall that the model is defined on the logit scale and thus, although relatively informative, a variance of 10 still represents a large enough value. As for the active treatment, we assume that the overall probability of contracting influenza is the same as the untreated population plus a decremental effect represented by the parameters δ_s.

These have an exchangeable structure defined in terms of the mean μ_δ, which represents the log-odds ratio for getting influenza under $t = 1$ (and against $t = 0$) and the variance σ_δ^2. Similarly to the evidence synthesis discussed above, we assign the following prior distributions

$$\mu_\gamma \sim \text{Normal}(0, v) \qquad \text{and} \qquad \sigma_\gamma \sim \text{Uniform}(0, 10).$$

Finally, we can combine the two evidence syntheses to derive an estimation for the probability of contracting influenza in the population treated with NIs. Since

$$\rho := \frac{p_1}{1 - p_1} \bigg/ \frac{p_0}{1 - p_0} = \exp(\mu_\delta)$$

represents the odds ratio of influenza (for $t = 1$ against $t = 0$), we can re-express the required probability using the identity

$$p_1 = \frac{\rho p_0/(1 - p_0)}{1 + \rho p_0/(1 - p_0)}.$$

Figure 5.7 shows a graphical representation of the two evidence syntheses described above, in terms of a DAG. As appears clear, the two evaluations are performed separately, but correlation among them is implied by the logical connection linking p_1 to p_0.

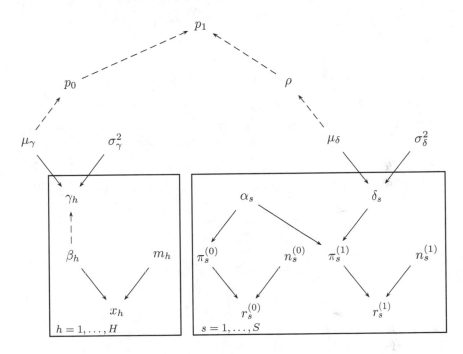

FIGURE 5.7
Graphical representation of the evidence syntheses in the model. In the graph, solid arrows indicate probabilistic links, while dashed arrows indicate logical dependence. H studies are used to investigate the overall population probability of being infected by influenza, p_0. A similar structure combines the information for the S studies investigating the effectiveness of NIs to derive an odds ratio, which is combined with the estimation of p_0 to provide an estimation of p_1, the probability of influenza in the scenario in which prophylactic treatment with NIs is made available.

According to the assumptions encoded in Figure 5.6 the measures of cost and effectiveness are then defined as

$$
\begin{aligned}
c_0 &= (1 - p_t)c^{\text{GP}} + p_t\left(c^{\text{GP}} + c^{\text{Inf}}\right) \\
c_1 &= (1 - p_t)\left(c^{\text{GP}} + c^{\text{NI}}\right) + p_t\left(c^{\text{GP}} + c^{\text{NI}} + c^{\text{Inf}}\right) \\
e_t &= lp_t.
\end{aligned}
$$

5.3.3 JAGS implementation

The model code is saved in the file EvSynth.txt and contains the following instructions. In the code, we use the notation r0[s] and r1[s] to indicate the variables $r_s^{(0)}$ and $r_s^{(1)}$, respectively. A similar notation is used for n0[s], n1[s], pi0[s] and pi1[s] (in place of $n_s^{(0)}$, $n_s^{(1)}$, $\pi_s^{(0)}$ and $\pi_s^{(1)}$).

```
model {
# Evidence synthesis on incidence of influenza in
#    the "healthy" adults population (t=0)
    for(h in 1:H) {
        x[h] ~ dbin(beta[h], m[h])
        logit(beta[h]) <- gamma[h]
        gamma[h] ~ dnorm(mu.gamma,tau.gamma)
    }

# Evidence synthesis for effectiveness of NIs (t=1 vs t=0)
    for (s in 1:S) {
        r0[s] ~ dbin(pi0[s],n0[s])
        r1[s] ~ dbin(pi1[s],n1[s])
        logit(pi0[s]) <- alpha[s]
        logit(pi1[s]) <- alpha[s]+delta[s]
        delta[s] ~ dnorm(mu.delta,tau.delta)
        alpha[s] ~ dnorm(0,0.00001)
    }

# Prior distributions
    mu.delta ~ dnorm(0,0.00001)
    mu.gamma ~ dnorm(0,0.00001)
    sigma.delta ~ dunif(0,10)
    tau.delta <- pow(sigma.delta,-2)
    sigma.gamma ~ dunif(0,10)
    tau.gamma <- pow(sigma.gamma,-2)

# Costs of influenza
    c.inf ~ dnorm(mu.inf,tau.inf)
# Length of time to recovery when infected by influenza
    l ~ dlnorm(mu.l,tau.l)

# Odds Ratio of influenza under treatment with NIs
    rho <- exp(mu.delta)
# Estimated probability of influenza in "healthy adults" for t=0
    p0 <- exp(mu.gamma)/(1+exp(mu.gamma))
# Estimated probability of influenza in "healthy adults" for t=1
    p1 <- (rho*p0/(1-p0))/(1+rho*p0/(1-p0))
}
```

The data pre-processing required in R involves the definition of the variables containing the observed data. We do this with the following code.

```
# Evidence synthesis on incidence of influenza
#    in healthy adults (under t=0)
x <- m <- numeric()
x <- c(0,6,5,6,25,18,14,3,27)
m <- c(23,241,159,137,519,298,137,24,132)
H <- length(x)

# Evidence synthesis on effectiveness of NIs vs placebo
r0 <- r1 <- n0 <- n1 <- numeric()
r0 <- c(34,40,9,19,6,34)
r1 <- c(11,7,3,3,3,4)
n0 <- c(554,423,144,268,251,462)
n1 <- c(553,414,144,268,252,493)
S <- length(r0)

# Data on costs
unit.cost.drug <- 2.4      # unit (daily) cost of NI
length.treat <- 6*7        # 6 weeks course of treatment
c.gp <- 19                 # cost of GP visit to prescribe NI
vat <- 1.175               # VAT @ 17.5%
c.ni <- unit.cost.drug*length.treat*vat

# Informative prior on cost of influenza
mu.inf <- 16.78            # mean cost of influenza episode
sigma.inf <- 2.34          # sd cost of influenza episode
tau.inf <- 1/sigma.inf^2   # precision cost of influenza episode

# Informative prior on length of influenza episodes
#   Computes mean, sd and precision time to recovery (log scale)
mu.l <- lognPar(8.2,sqrt(2))$mulog
sigma.l <- lognPar(8.2,sqrt(2))$sigmalog
tau.l <- 1/sigma.l^2
```

First we define the vectors x and m in which we put the observed values, available in Cooper et al. (2004). For simplicity, the variable H is computed, rather than inputed, by assigning it the value of the length of the vector x (of course, it would make no difference whatsoever if we actually assigned it a value, e.g. H <- 9). A similar reasoning applies to the second evidence synthesis, for which data are again available from the original study.

We then compute the cost of treatment with NIs for a six-week course and define the parameters for the distribution of influenza-related costs. Since these are set on the natural scale, we can simply define the values for the mean and standard deviation and then compute the precision (required by JAGS/BUGS) as the reciprocal of the variance.

Finally, we use the function lognPar (cfr. §4.7) to compute the parameters of the distribution of the length of time with influenza, which is modelled on the log scale.

The model can now be run calling the function JAGS, which we do using the following code.

```
library(R2jags)
dataJags <- list("S","H","r0","r1","n0","n1","x","m",
                 "mu.inf","tau.inf","mu.l","tau.l")
filein <- "EvSynth.txt"
params <- c("p0","p1","rho","l","c.inf","alpha","delta","gamma")
inits <- function(){
  list(alpha=rnorm(S,0,1),delta=rnorm(S,0,1),mu.delta=rnorm(1),
       sigma.delta=runif(1),gamma=rnorm(H,0,1),mu.gamma=rnorm(1),
       sigma.gamma=runif(1),c.inf=rnorm(1),l=runif(1))
}


n.iter <- 10000
n.burnin <- 5000
n.thin <- floor((n.iter-n.burnin)/500)
es <- jags(dataJags,inits,params,model.file=filein,
    n.chains=2, n.iter, n.burnin, n.thin, DIC=TRUE)
print(es,digits=3,intervals=c(0.025, 0.975))
attach.bugs(es$BUGSoutput)
```

The code is pretty straightforward and the only noteworthy aspect is that we initialise the variable l using a Uniform distribution on $(0; 1)$. This gives a reasonable value, given that this variable has a logNormal distribution. Of course, other choices are possible, but this has not a crucial impact on the final convergence of the model.

The results are then printed and attached to the R workspace. As is possible to see from the summary table, while autocorrelation seems present for some of the variables, convergence is generally reached satisfactorily, especially for the parameters of main interest in the cost-effectiveness analysis $\theta = (p_0, p_1, l, c_{inf})$.

```
Inference for Bugs model at "EvSynth.txt", fit using jags,
 2 chains, each with 20000 iterations (first 10000 discarded),
 n.thin = 20, n.sims = 1000 iterations saved
          mu.vect sd.vect   2.5%   97.5% Rhat n.eff
alpha[1]   -2.695   0.181 -3.068  -2.363 1.012   120
alpha[2]   -2.293   0.158 -2.617  -1.997 1.000  1000
alpha[3]   -2.641   0.307 -3.261  -2.068 1.001  1000
alpha[4]   -2.661   0.233 -3.170  -2.242 1.008   200
alpha[5]   -3.609   0.374 -4.439  -2.954 1.007  1000
alpha[6]   -2.587   0.167 -2.930  -2.268 1.001  1000
```

```
c.inf        16.825   2.292 12.389   21.469 1.002    980
delta[1]     -1.408   0.313 -1.977   -0.763 1.019     82
delta[2]     -1.715   0.328 -2.439   -1.113 1.021    150
delta[3]     -1.493   0.409 -2.238   -0.568 1.003    510
delta[4]     -1.706   0.379 -2.543   -0.972 1.012    800
delta[5]     -1.350   0.522 -2.152   -0.094 1.047     41
delta[6]     -1.874   0.379 -2.754   -1.261 1.001   1000
gamma[1]     -3.549   0.900 -5.636   -2.146 1.001   1000
gamma[2]     -3.561   0.369 -4.436   -2.926 1.001   1000
gamma[3]     -3.344   0.406 -4.257   -2.653 1.001   1000
gamma[4]     -3.070   0.375 -3.831   -2.385 1.011    280
gamma[5]     -2.979   0.204 -3.402   -2.596 1.000   1000
gamma[6]     -2.771   0.236 -3.248   -2.328 1.007   1000
gamma[7]     -2.283   0.282 -2.846   -1.748 1.007    250
gamma[8]     -2.344   0.583 -3.505   -1.221 1.000   1000
gamma[9]     -1.474   0.225 -1.905   -1.026 1.000   1000
l             8.191   1.388  5.760   11.284 1.001   1000
p1            0.060   0.022  0.028    0.108 1.002    870
p2            0.014   0.009  0.005    0.036 1.009    180
rho           0.225   0.114  0.109    0.508 1.017    190
deviance    102.128   5.865 92.571  114.949 1.003    520
```

For each parameter, n.eff is a crude measure of effective sample size, and Rhat is the potential scale reduction factor (at convergence, Rhat=1).

DIC info (using the rule, pD = var(deviance)/2)
pD = 17.2 and DIC = 119.3
DIC is an estimate of expected predictive error (lower deviance is better).

5.3.4 Cost-effectiveness analysis

Before we can run the economic analysis, we now need to define the variables of cost and effectiveness, which we do with the following R code and in accordance with the model structure presented above.

```
# Defines the variables of cost and effectiveness
c <- e <- matrix(NA,n.sims,2)
c[,1] <- (1-p1)*(c.gp) + p1*(c.gp+c.inf)
c[,2] <- (1-p2)*(c.gp+c.ni) + p2*(c.gp+c.ni+c.inf)
e[,1] <- -l*p1
e[,2] <- -l*p2
```

These variables can be then used to run the function bcea.

```
# Runs the economic analysis
library(BCEA)
treats <- c("status quo","prophylaxis with NIs")
m <- bcea(e,c,ref=2,treats,Kmax=10000)
```

The command summary(m) produces a summary table with the results of the economic evaluation.

```
Cost-effectiveness analysis summary

Reference intervention: prophylaxis with NIs
Comparator intervention: status quo

Optimal decision: choose status quo for k<320 and prophylaxis with NIs for k>=320


Analysis for willingness to pay parameter k = 10000

                        Expected utility
status quo                   -4904.5
prophylaxis with NIs         -1285.5


                                    EIB  CEAC   ICER
prophylaxis with NIs vs status quo 3619 0.994 314.92

Optimal intervention (max expected utility) for k=10000: prophylaxis with NIs

EVPI 3.7043
```

The cost-effectiveness of prophylactic NIs seems to be proved as the ICER is very small and there does not seem to be much uncertainty attached to this result. The CEAC is nearly 1 for k as low as £10 000 (which is nearly half of the cost-effectiveness treshold usually recommended by NICE). Similarly, the EVPI is very low and it reaches the value of £18 at the break-even point.

5.4   Markov models

One simple way of describing a decision problem consists in using *decision trees* (DTs), i.e. a graphical structure combined with conditional probability and utility measures (e.g. costs or quality of life indicators) associated with different decisions.

An example of DT is given in Figure 5.8. The root of the tree (the leftmost part in the graph) is a decision node (depicted as a square), which is associated with several *branches*, representing the possible interventions. Each path is characterised by random nodes (depicted as a circles). One of the possible consequences (the branches departing from the random nodes) will obtain in the future, according to the probability distribution characterising the problem. This will lead to the *leaf* (depicted as a diamond), which is the final part of the tree and is associated with the utility $u(y, t)$ of a specific path (consequence). The computation of the expected utility is made by weighing the utility functions attached to each leaf by these probabilities. This process is referred to as *averaging and folding back*.

While DTs are easy to construct and analyse, they typically become intractable when the number of possible decisions or random consequences increases beyond very small numbers. Moreover, to model recurrent situations,

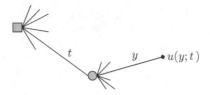

FIGURE 5.8
An example of a decision tree. Decision nodes are represented by squares, while random nodes are represented as circles. Finally, utility nodes are depicted by diamonds. The tree describes the possible path characterising decision, consequences and utilities. For example, the selection of treatment t leads to the realisation of the random consequence y, which is in turns associated with a utility $u(y,t)$.

where decisions and random events occur at several time points, is generally quite difficult in a DT.

This is relevant when the main objective of the economic evaluation is to produce an estimation of the clinical pathway of a particular disease (which is often the case, particularly when dealing with decision analytic models). Thus, in order to model clinical decision problems in a realistic way it is necessary to move to a more advanced methodology.

One such possible extension, which is increasingly often used in health economic evaluations, is represented by *Markov models* (Sonneberg and Beck, 1993; Briggs and Sculpher, 1998; Hunnink and Glasziou, 2001; Parmigiani, 2002b; Spiegelhalter and Best, 2003; Spiegelhalter et al., 2004; Rushby and Cairns, 2005; Briggs et al., 2006).

In a Markov model (MM), the natural history of the disease under study is represented by patients' movements (or, to use a more technical term, *transitions*) over time and a finite (and usually discrete) set of *states* that are assumed to be representative of the management of the disease. Usually, time is modelled through a set of discrete *cycles* (e.g. years).

The basic characteristics of MMs are the following:

A1 at each time point, each individual in the reference population can be in one and only one of the states used to represent the clinical problem in its entirety. In other words, the states are assumed to be *exhaustive* and *mutually exclusive*.

A2 At the end of each cycle, each individual can move from the state in which they currently are to one of the other states. In particular, the movements are governed by a set of suitable *transition probabilities*, which are assumed to be independent on the path that has led a given individual to the current state (a condition referred to as *Markov property*, which we discuss in §5.4.5). However, these transition probabilities can depend on the time point or other risk factors.

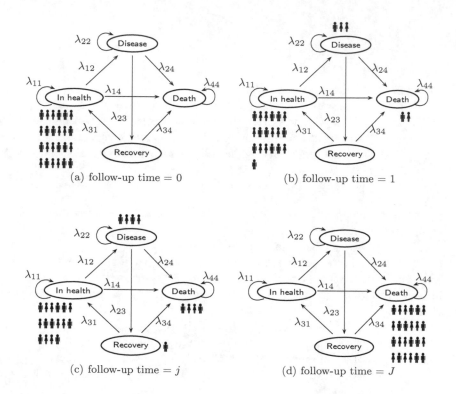

FIGURE 5.9
A graphical representation of a Markov model. In panel (a), the structure is defined in terms of transition probabilities. Arrows connecting two nodes indicate that it is possible to move from the node where the arrow originates to the one which is reached by it. The corresponding transition probability is defined by the random quantity $\lambda_{ss'}$. Typically, at the start of the "virtual" follow-up, all patients are assumed to be in the state In health. In panel (b), the patients start to move from the healthy state towards the others, according to the transition probabilities. The follow-up continues in panel (c), where fewer patients are healthy and more are progressing towards the other states. Eventually, at the final time of the follow-up all patients have reached the state Death.

Figure 5.9 shows an example of Markov model. In this simple example, we assume that patients can be either healthy, affected by the disease under study, recovering from the disease, or dead. No other clinical state is assumed to be relevant and therefore these four states are considered to be fully representative of the clinical pathways that the patients can experience.

The arrows connecting two nodes (i.e. clinical states) indicate that it is possible to move from the node where the arrow originates to the one which is reached by it. For example, patients who at time j are in the state In health, can either remain healthy, move to the state Disease, or die (i.e. move to Death), at the next time point $(j + 1)$.

These movements are controlled by a corresponding transition probability, defined for each pair of states (s, s') by the random quantity $\lambda_{ss'}$. The absence of an arrow connecting two nodes encodes the assumption that patients cannot move between them. For example, because they have not got the disease yet, patients who find themselves in the state In health cannot go directly to the state Recovery.

Once a suitable structure is defined to describe the relationships between the clinical states and the transition probabilities are estimated, it is possible to use the MM to simulate the possible outcomes for a "virtual" cohort of patients to whom a given intervention t is applied. In other words, the MM is run to obtain a simulation of a large number of "possible futures" for a given cohort, under the probabilistic assumptions. These simulations can be used to derive a complete (posterior) probability distribution of the possible outcomes, which can then be summarised (e.g. by taking the average values of costs and measures of effectiveness over the large number of simulations).

For example, in Figure 5.9 we consider a cohort formed by 24 individuals. At the beginning of observation, all patients are assumed to be healthy, as shown in panel (a).

At the next time period, shown in panel (b), the patients start to move according to the transition probabilities. For example, we can expect three members of the cohort to become ill and two to die. Of course, at this point in time, no patient can find themselves in the Recovery state, since no one was diseased at the previous time.

As the follow-up continues, patients keep moving among the states. For example, patients who were in the state Disease at the previous time can either remain in that state, proceed to Recovery, or die. In panel (c) there are now four patients in the Disease state; of the three present at the previous time, one has moved to the state of Recovery, while there are now four patients who are dead.

If the virtual follow-up is long enough, eventually all patients move to the state Death. This situation is shown in panel (d). Of course, individuals cannot move away from the state Death. A clinical state with such a characteristic is termed an *absorbent* state.

Formally, a *discrete state/discrete time* MM considers J cycles and S possible states. At the beginning of the first cycle $j = 1$, the probability distribution of the states is represented by a vector $\boldsymbol{\pi}_1 = (\pi_{11}, \ldots \pi_{1S})$, whose generic element π_{1s} represents the probability that at time $j = 1$ a random individual from the population is in state s.

The transition probabilities can be arranged in a matrix $\mathbf{\Lambda}_j$, whose generic element $\lambda_{jss'}$ represents the probability of a transition from state s to state s' between cycles $(j-1)$ and j. By means of this construction, we can retrieve a recursive relationship that holds for each $j > 1$ and allows us to compute the probability distribution of the states at any time point

$$\boldsymbol{\pi}_j = \boldsymbol{\pi}_{j-1} \times \mathbf{\Lambda}_j. \tag{5.8}$$

Sometimes, it is reasonable to assume that the matrix $\mathbf{\Lambda}_j$ does not depend on time, which generally simplifies the calculations. In that case, in order to estimate the probability distributions of the states at each time j it is only necessary to know the initial distribution $\boldsymbol{\pi}_1$ and the constant transition matrix $\mathbf{\Lambda}$.

Often, instead of the probability distribution of the states $\boldsymbol{\pi}_j$, it is useful to consider the absolute number of patients sojourning in each state, which we indicate as $\mathbf{m}_j = (m_{j1} \ldots, m_{jS})$, where the generic element m_{js} represents the total number of patients in state s at time j. It is easy to re-express (5.8) as

$$\mathbf{m}_j = \mathbf{m}_{j-1} \times \mathbf{\Lambda}_j. \tag{5.9}$$

The costs and utilities associated with each clinical state can be multiplied by the number of patients present at each time point in each state, in order to estimate the relevant economic summaries. In general, because the time horizon of a MM is large, it is necessary to discount the measures of cost and effectiveness (cfr. §1.5).

In summary, the steps required to perform an economic analysis based on a MM are the following.

i. Define a structure to represent the relevant clinical states and the relationships among them in terms of possible transitions.

ii. Estimate the relevant transition probabilities that form the transition matrices $\mathbf{\Lambda}_j$.

iii. Run the MM to simulate a set of possible future outcomes, recording both costs and clinical benefits associated with each state at each time point.

iv. Perform the economic analysis, applying discounting if the time horizon is longer than one year.

Step *ii.* represents the main inferential task related to the execution of the MM. Sometimes it is possible to directly estimate the elements of the matrices $\mathbf{\Lambda}_j$ using observed data on the relevant transitions. These might be obtained for example by RCTs or observational studies in which a set of individuals is followed up for a (usually limited) period of time (cfr. §5.4.1).

Alternatively, when individual data on the observed transitions are not available, it is possible to build a set of deterministic relationships that define the elements $\lambda_{jss'}$ in terms of suitable parameters $\boldsymbol{\theta}$, which become the objective of the modelling procedure, perhaps by means of a suitable evidence synthesis. Once the uncertainty on $\boldsymbol{\theta}$ is described (e.g. by means of a posterior distribution), it is possible to compute the implied distributions for $\boldsymbol{\Lambda}_j$ and proceed with steps *iii.* and *iv.* to produce the required economic evaluation. An example of this strategy is discussed in §5.4.6.

5.4.1   Example: Markov model for the treatment of asthma

We consider a well known example in the health economic literature, originally described in Price and Briggs (2002) and Briggs et al. (2003).

The interest is in modelling the cost-effectiveness of two alternative treatments for asthma, a common chronic-episodic disease characterised by acute, symptomatic episodes of varying severity. Clinical symptoms (including wheezing and coughing) are usually accompanied by reduced lung functions.

Asthma exacerbations have an economic impact because they can require intervention by a health care professional, which leads to extra costs incurred. Although relatively rare, hospitalisations are the most relevant outcome because of their high cost. The clinical setting of an exacerbation is also an indicator of the severity of the event. When patients are not experiencing moderate or severe exacerbations at any given point in time, they are defined to be either adequately controlled or symptomatic at a level that does not require intervention by a health care professional.

The original model assumes $S = 5$ distinct and mutually exclusive health states: *successfully treated week* (STW, which we code as $s = 1$), indicating the appropriate asthma control; *unsuccessfully treated week* (UTW, $s = 2$), indicating suboptimal control; *primary care-managed exacerbation* (Pex, $s = 3$); *hospital-managed exacerbation* (Hex, $s = 4$); and *treatment failure* (TF, $s = 5$). TF indicates the point at which patients discontinued the treatment under study and entered a "usual-care" pattern of asthma management.

Figure 5.4.1 shows the Markov model representation of the problem. Note that the state TF is considered to be an absorbent state: once patients reach it, then they remain in that condition and it is not possible to move back to one of the other clinical states.

The two competing treatments are $t = 0$: Fluticasone proprionate alone with a dosage of $100\mu g$ (FP) and; $t = 1$: a combination of Salmeterol $50\mu g$ and Fluticasone proprionate $100\mu g$ (SFC), which represents the intervention whose cost-effectiveness is being evaluated.

The model is informed by data observed in a $J = 12$ week RCT. For each treatment, we define the variable $r_{ss'}^{(t)}$ to indicate the observed total number of transitions from state s to state s' $(s, s' = 1, \ldots, S)$ from one week to the next, aggregating over all J weeks. Similarly, we indicate the total number of transitions out of a generic state s as $n_s^{(t)}$. Table 5.2 shows the observed values for both treatments.

The observed data can be used to estimate the transition probabilities $\lambda_{ss'}^{(t)}$,

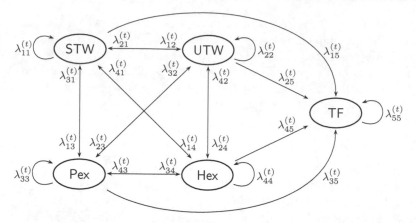

FIGURE 5.10

Graphical representation of the treatment of asthma in terms of a Markov model. Connections with double arrows indicate that it is possible to move from state s to state s' *and* from state s' to state s. Each possible transition is associated with a suitable probability $\lambda_{ss'}^{(t)}$, specific to each intervention t.

TABLE 5.2

Observed number of transitions among the clinical states. For each intervention t, the entries in the main part of the tables indicate $r_{ss'}^{(t)}$, the total number of observed transitions from state s in week j to state s' in week $(j+1)$, aggregated over all J weeks. The row totals $n_s^{(t)}$ (included in the final column of the table) indicate the total number of transitions out of state s

Intervention $t=0$		STW	UTW	Hex	Pex	TF	Total $n_s^{(0)}$
STW	$(s=1)$	66	32	0	0	2	100
UTW	$(s=2)$	42	752	0	5	20	819
Pex	$(s=3)$	0	4	0	1	0	5
Hex	$(s=4)$	0	0	0	0	0	0
TF	$(s=5)$	0	0	0	0	156	156

Intervention $t=1$		STW	UTW	Hex	Pex	TF	Total $n_s^{(1)}$
STW	$(s=1)$	210	60	0	1	1	272
UTW	$(s=2)$	88	641	0	4	13	746
Pex	$(s=3)$	1	0	0	0	1	2
Hex	$(s=4)$	0	0	0	0	0	0
TF	$(s=5)$	0	0	0	0	81	81

which can be arranged in the transition matrix

$$
\Lambda^{(t)} = \begin{pmatrix}
\lambda_{11}^{(t)} & \lambda_{12}^{(t)} & \cdots & \lambda_{1S}^{(t)} \\
\lambda_{21}^{(t)} & \lambda_{22}^{(t)} & \cdots & \lambda_{2S}^{(t)} \\
\vdots & \vdots & \ddots & \vdots \\
\lambda_{S1}^{(t)} & \lambda_{S2}^{(t)} & \cdots & \lambda_{SS}^{(t)}
\end{pmatrix}.
$$

These in turn characterise the follow-up of the virtual cohort used to perform the economic analysis. In particular, we assume that at time $j = 1$, all $N^{(t)}$ patients are in the state STW.

By simply extending (5.9), we can compute the number of patients who at time $j + 1$ are in state s as

$$
\begin{aligned}
m_{(j+1)s}^{(t)} &= m_{j1}^{(t)}\lambda_{1s}^{(t)} + m_{j2}^{(t)}\lambda_{2s}^{(t)} + m_{j3}^{(t)}\lambda_{3s}^{(t)} + m_{j4}^{(t)}\lambda_{4s}^{(t)} + m_{j5}^{(t)}\lambda_{5s}^{(t)} \\
&= \sum_{s'=1}^{S} m_{js'}^{(t)}\lambda_{s's}^{(t)}.
\end{aligned}
\tag{5.10}
$$

In this particular case, the transition matrix $\Lambda^{(t)}$ is supposed independent on time j. This is reasonable, also in consideration of the short time horizon considered in this analysis. As suggested earlier, in other circumstances this might not be appropriate and therefore the matrix $\Lambda^{(t)}$ should be modelled as a function of the index j.

We can use the vectors $\mathbf{m}_j^{(t)}$ to characterise the measures of cost and benefit associated with each treatment. For instance, we assume that patients who at any time are in one of the first four states are associated with a fixed cost (Price and Briggs, 2002), shown in Table 5.3.

TABLE 5.3
Fixed cost of transition in states $s = 1, \ldots, 4$ for each treatment. The entries of the table represent the values $c_s^{(t)}$. Source: Price and Briggs (2002)

Intervention	STW: $c_1^{(t)}$	UTW: $c_2^{(t)}$	Pex: $c_3^{(t)}$	Hex: $c_4^{(t)}$
$t = 0$	£2.38	£2.38	£95.21	£1815.58
$t = 1$	£7.96	£7.96	£100.79	£1821.17

As for the absorbent state TP, the associated cost is computed as a weighted average of the cost produced by patients in the other states under the status quo ($t = 0$), where the weights are given by the total number of individuals present in each

$$
c_{5j} = \frac{\displaystyle\sum_{s=1}^{4} m_{js}^{(0)} c_s^{(0)}}{\displaystyle\sum_{s=1}^{4} m_{js}^{(0)}}.
\tag{5.11}
$$

Slightly abusing the notation, we can then define the total cost associated with each treatment as

$$
c_t = \sum_{j=1}^{J} m_{jS}^{(t)} c_{5j} + \sum_{j=1}^{J}\sum_{s=1}^{S-1} m_{js}^{(t)} c_{sj}^{(t)}.
$$

As for the benefits, we follow Briggs et al. (2003) and consider the total number of weeks that the patients spend in the STW state, which is computed as

$$e_t = \sum_{j=1}^{J} m_{j1}^{(t)}.$$

Notice that because the time horizon is short (only 12 weeks), we do not apply discounting to the results observed over time in the virtual follow up.

5.4.2   Model description

For each state s, we can arrange the overall observed number of transitions in a vector $\mathbf{r}_s^{(t)} = \left(r_{s1}^{(t)}, \ldots, r_{sS}^{(t)} \right)$. In general, we can model these vectors using a Multinomial distribution

$$\mathbf{r}_s^{(t)} \mid \boldsymbol{\lambda}_s^{(t)} \sim \text{Multinomial} \left(\boldsymbol{\lambda}_s^{(t)}, n_s^{(t)} \right)$$

$$= \frac{n_s^{(t)}!}{r_{s1}^{(t)}! \cdots r_{sS}^{(t)}!} \lambda_{s1}^{(t)r_{s1}^{(t)}} \cdots \lambda_{sS}^{(t)r_{sS}^{(t)}}$$

as a function of a set of parameters $\boldsymbol{\lambda}_s^{(t)} = \left(\lambda_{s1}^{(t)}, \ldots, \lambda_{sS}^{(t)} \right)$, with the constraint that $\sum_{s'=1}^{S} \lambda_{ss'}^{(t)} = 1$. The vectors $\boldsymbol{\lambda}_s^{(t)}$ include the transition probabilities, while $n_s^{(t)} = \sum_{s'=1}^{S} r_{ss'}^{(t)}$ is the sample size.

A convenient prior distribution to be associated with $\boldsymbol{\lambda}_s^{(t)}$ is represented by the Dirichlet model

$$\boldsymbol{\lambda}_s^{(t)} \mid \boldsymbol{\alpha}^{(t)} \sim \text{Dirichlet} \left(\alpha_1^{(t)}, \ldots, \alpha_S^{(t)} \right) \tag{5.12}$$

$$= \frac{\Gamma \left(\alpha_1^{(t)} + \ldots + \alpha_S^{(t)} \right)}{\Gamma \left(\alpha_1^{(t)} \right) \cdots \Gamma \left(\alpha_S^{(t)} \right)} \lambda_{s1}^{(t)(\alpha_1^{(t)}-1)} \cdots \lambda_{sS}^{(t)(\alpha_S^{(t)}-1)}$$

where $\boldsymbol{\alpha}^{(t)} = \left(\alpha_1^{(t)}, \ldots, \alpha_S^{(t)} \right)$ is a vector of hyper-parameters.

The Multinomial-Dirichlet model described above can be thought of as a multivariate generalisation of the conjugate Binomial-Beta model discussed in §2.4.2. Intuitively, we can think of $\sum_{s=1}^{S} \alpha_s^{(t)}$ as a prior sample size; the value of each element $\alpha_s^{(t)}$ is proportional to the expected probability $\lambda_{ss'}^{(t)}$. Consequently, assuming that all the elements in $\boldsymbol{\alpha}^{(t)}$ are equivalent to some pre-specified scale value $\phi^{(t)}$, encodes the assumption that all the transitions from state s are equally likely. For the sake of simplicity, for all t we set $\phi^{(t)} = 1$ (which amounts to assuming a relatively vague prior), but of course sensitivity to this choice should be explicitly analysed.

In the current example, we can simplify the above model by noting the following aspects. First, for both interventions, there are no transitions from the state Hex in the observed data. Thus, although it is necessary to estimate the transition probabilities $\boldsymbol{\lambda}_4^{(t)}$ to construct the MM, it does not make sense to build an observational model for $\mathbf{r}_4^{(t)}$. Within the Bayesian context, this is not a problem, because we can use a subjective prior to model $\boldsymbol{\lambda}_4^{(t)}$, based for example on the relevant expert knowledge.

Second, because by definition the state TP is absorbent, we do not need to estimate the associated transition probabilities, which are logically defined as $\boldsymbol{\lambda}_5^{(t)} = (0,0,0,0,1)$.

Consequently, the model comprises the following three sub-models.

m1. For $s = 1, 2, 3$: $\mathbf{r}_s^{(t)} \mid \boldsymbol{\lambda}_s^{(t)} \sim \text{Multinomial}\left(\boldsymbol{\lambda}_s^{(t)}, n_s^{(t)}\right)$ and

$$\boldsymbol{\lambda}_s^{(t)} \mid \boldsymbol{\alpha}^{(t)} \sim \text{Dirichlet}\left(\alpha_1^{(t)}, \ldots, \alpha_S^{(t)}\right).$$

m2. For $s = 4$: $\boldsymbol{\lambda}_s^{(t)} \mid \boldsymbol{\alpha}^{(t)} \sim \text{Dirichlet}\left(\alpha_1^{(t)}, \ldots, \alpha_S^{(t)}\right).$

m3. For $s = 5$: $\boldsymbol{\lambda}_s^{(t)} = (0,0,0,0,1).$

5.4.3   JAGS implementation

We code the model described above using the following specification

```
model {
# m1. Multinomial distribution for r, Dirichlet prior for lambda
    for(s in 1:3){
        r.0[s,1:S] ~ dmulti(lambda.0[s,1:S], n.0[s])
        r.1[s,1:S] ~ dmulti(lambda.1[s,1:S], n.1[s])
        lambda.0[s,1:S] ~ ddirch(alpha.0[1:S])
        lambda.1[s,1:S] ~ ddirch(alpha.1[1:S])
    }

# m2. Dirichlet prior for the non-observed state (Hex)
    lambda.0[4,1:S] ~ ddirch(alpha.0[1:S])
    lambda.1[4,1:S] ~ ddirch(alpha.1[1:S])

# m3. Deterministic values for the absorbent state (TP)
    for (s in 1:4) {
        lambda.0[S,s] <- 0
        lambda.1[S,s] <- 0
    }
    lambda.0[S,S] <- 1
    lambda.1[S,S] <- 1
}
```

which we save in the file MarkovModel1.txt.

The relevant data can be loaded in R by using the following code.

```
S <- 5                        # number of states
J <- 12                       # number of time points
r.0 <- (matrix(c(             # observed cases for t=0
  66,32,0,0,2,
  42,752,0,5,20,
  0,4,0,1,0),c(3,S),byrow=TRUE)
r.1 <- (matrix(c(             # observed cases for t=1
  210,60,0,1,1,
  88,641,0,4,13,
  1,0,0,0,1),c(3,S),byrow=TRUE)
n.0 <- apply(r.0,1,sum)       # number of patients in
n.1 <- apply(r.1,1,sum)       #   each state for t=0,1
scale <- 1                    # level of informativeness for
alpha.0 <- alpha.1 <- rep(scale,S) #   the Dirichlet prior
```

In line with the discussion above, we only include the data on the observed transitions for $s = 1, 2, 3$. In particular, the values are entered in matrix form (i.e. S values for each of the 3 relevant states). In the absence of substantial knowledge on the possible transitions off the state Hex, we use the same flat prior for all the vectors $\boldsymbol{\lambda}_s^{(t)}$. Obviously, because there are no data for $\mathbf{r}_4^{(t)}$, the resulting posteriors for $\boldsymbol{\lambda}_4^{(t)}$ will be close to Uniform distributions, assigning approximately $1/S$ of the probability to each state.

We then prepare the call to the function jags to actually run the model using the following code.

```
library(R2jags)
dataJags <- list("n.0","n.1","r.0","r.1","alpha.0","alpha.1","S")
filein <- "MarkovModel1.txt"
params <- c("lambda.0","lambda.1")
inits <- function(){
    temp.0 <- matrix(rgamma(4*S,scale,1),4,S)
    sum.temp.0 <- apply(temp.0,1,sum)
    mat.0 <- temp.0/sum.temp.0
    temp.1 <- matrix(rgamma(4*S,scale,1),4,S)
    sum.temp.1 <- apply(temp.1,1,sum)
    mat.1 <- temp.1/sum.temp.1
    list(lambda.0=rbind(mat.0,rep(NA,S)),
         lambda.1=rbind(mat.1,rep(NA,S))
    )
}

n.iter <- 10000
n.burnin <- 5000
n.thin <- floor((n.iter-n.burnin)/500)
mm1 <- jags(dataJags,inits,params,model.file=filein,
    n.chains=2, n.iter, n.burnin, n.thin, DIC=TRUE)
```

```
print(mm1,digits=3,intervals=c(0.025, 0.975))
attach.bugs(mm1$BUGSoutput)
```

The most interesting part of the code consists of the definition of the inits. The only random variables in the model are the vectors $\boldsymbol{\lambda}_s^{(t)}$ and the easiest option is to initialise them using random draws from a Dirichlet distribution (which would ensure reasonable values).

In order to do this, we can use a well known result of standard probability calculus. For each $s = 1, \ldots, 4$, first we simulate a vector of S values obtained independently using a Gamma distribution with parameters $(\boldsymbol{\alpha}^{(t)}, 1)$. The results are saved in a matrices temp.0 and temp.1.

These are then rescaled to ensure that each simulated value is in the interval $[0; 1]$ and that their sum is 1. We do so by dividing each row of the two matrices by its total, which we have computed in the vectors sum.temp.0 and sum.temp.1. The results are saved in the matrices mat.0 and mat.1.

Finally, we account for the fact that the vectors $\boldsymbol{\lambda}_5^{(t)}$ cannot be initialised (given their deterministic nature) by appending a vector of S NA values to mat.0 and mat.1.

The model can then be run and the posterior distributions for the transition matrix $\boldsymbol{\Lambda}^{(t)}$ saved and attached to the R workspace.

5.4.4 Cost-effectiveness analysis

Once the posterior distribution of the transition probabilities has been estimated, we can define and run the MM. In theory, we can code the relevant relationships directly in the JAGS/BUGS code. However, it is in general more effective to perform this step in R, to speed up the execution of the MCMC procedure.

```
# Markov model
m.0 <- m.1 <- array(NA,c(n.sims,S,(J+1)))
  for (s in 1:S){                    # Assumes only 1 patient
     m.0[,s,1] <- c(1,0,0,0,0)       #  initially in the state
     m.1[,s,1] <- c(1,0,0,0,0)       #  'In health'
}

for (i in 1:n.sims) {
    for (j in 2:(J+1)){
       for (s in 1:S){
          m.0[i,s,j] <- sum(m.0[i,,j-1]*lambda.0[i,,s])
          m.1[i,s,j] <- sum(m.1[i,,j-1]*lambda.1[i,,s])
       }
    }
}
```

First, we define two vectors m.0 and m.1 in which we will store the estimated number of people in each of the states and at each time. The vectors represent $\mathbf{m}_j^{(0)}$ and $\mathbf{m}_j^{(1)}$, respectively. Then, we need to initialise them, i.e. define the distribution of patients at time $j = 1$. In this particular instance, we assume that we are following up just one patient, who is initially healthy. Of course, this is not always the case, but it is easy to modify the code above to account for different situations.

Finally, we program the recursive relationship (5.10) to compute the number of patients in each state for any time in the follow-up. The R notation follows closely the algebraic form of this expression and thus should be quite obvious. Notice that because time $j = 1$ is just the initialisation point, we run the MM for $(J+1)$ times, which will give an overall follow-up of J time points.

Figure 5.11 shows the results of the MM in terms of the average proportion of patients in each state and at each of the virtual follow-up points.

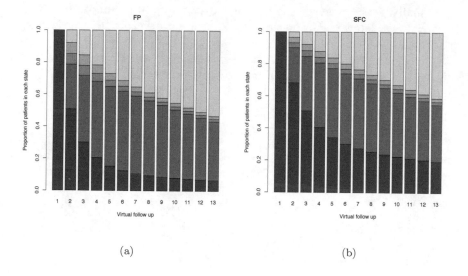

FIGURE 5.11
Simulation of the cohort of patients. Panel (a) shows the result for $t = 0$ (FP), while panel (b) shows the results for $t = 1$ (SFC). The darker bar indicates STW, while increasingly lighter bars are UTW, Pex, Hex and TF (the lightest shade of grey). On average, $t = 1$ seems to produce a greater proportion of people that remain in the state STW and a smaller proportion of patients ending up in the least favourable state, TF.

At the end of the `for` loop, the R workspace contains two arrays `m.0` and `m.1`, each of dimension `(n.sims, J+1, S)`, which can be used to compute the variables of costs and benefits. We do so using the following code.

```
# Unit costs for the non-absorbent states
```

```
c.0 <- c(2.38,2.38,1815.58,95.21)
c.1 <- c(7.96,7.96,1821.17,100.79)

# Computes total weekly costs
cost0 <- cost1 <- matrix(0,n.sims,J)
for (i in 1:n.sims){
    for (j in 2:(J+1)){
        c5[j] <- (c.0%*%m.0[i,1:(S-1),j])/sum(m.0[i,1:(S-1),j])
        cost0[i,j-1] <- m.0[i,S,j]*c5[j] + c.0%*%m.0[i,1:(S-1),j]
        cost1[i,j-1] <- m.1[i,S,j]*c5[j] + c.1%*%m.1[i,1:(S-1),j]
    }
}
```

First, we define the unit cost associated with each of the first four states. Then we define two matrices cost.0 and cost.1, each of dimension (n.sims, J) and originally filled with 0 values. For each time point in the follow up j, we first compute the cost of the state TP, according to (5.11).

Here, the R notation %*% codifies the *inner product* between the elements of two vectors. Thus the command

```
c.0%*%m.0[i,1:(S-1),j]
```

is equivalent to writing

```
c.0[1]*m.0[i,1,j] + c.0[2]*m.0[i,2,j] + ... + c.0[S-1]*m.0[i,S-1,j]
```

Because in the current example the time horizon is limited, there is no need to discount costs and clinical benefits. However, if discounting were a relevant issue, it could easily be applied, for example using the following code.

```
## Generic code to apply discount
# Defines the discount RATE for costs and benefits
delta.c <- 0.035      # discount rate for costs (3.5%)
delta.b <- 0.035      # discount rate for benefits (3.5%)

# Defines the discount FACTORS for each time point
disc.b <- disc.c <- numeric()
disc.b[1] <- disc.c[1] <- 1   # ie no discount at time j=1
for (j in 2:J) {
    disc.b[j] <- (1+delta.b)^(j-1)
    disc.c[j] <- (1+delta.c)^(j-1)
}

# Computes the discounted costs and effects
disc.cost0 <- disc.eff0 <- matrix(NA,n.sims,J)
disc.cost1 <- disc.eff1 <- matrix(NA,n.sims,J)
for (j in 1:J) {
```

```
    disc.cost0[,j] <- cost0[,j]/disc.c[j]
    disc.cost1[,j] <- cost1[,j]/disc.c[j]
    disc.eff0[,j] <- m.0[,1,j]/disc.b[j]
    disc.eff1[,j] <- m.1[,1,j]/disc.b[j]
}
```

First, the discount rates for costs and benefits are defined in the variables delta.c and delta.b. In this example we set them to 3.5% for both the quantities of interest, in line with the discussion of §1.5. Then, for each time point, we compute the discount factor and finally we compute the ratio of the original costs and benefits to the discount factors, as in (1.1). Of course, setting delta.b = delta.c = 0 would imply no discounting at all.

The analysis can be completed by aggregating the costs over the time points, which can be done in R typing the following commands (and if discount was applied, the variables cost0, cost1, m.0[,1,] and m.1[,1,] would be replaced by disc.cost0, disc.cost1, disc.eff0 and disc.eff1, respectively).

```
# Sums across all time points and creates the matrices of costs
c <- matrix(NA,n.sims,2)
c[,1] <- apply(cost0,1,sum)
c[,2] <- apply(cost1,1,sum)

# Effectiveness: total weeks in STW (state s=1)
e <- matrix(NA,n.sims,2)
e[,1] <- apply(m.0[,1,],1,sum)
e[,2] <- apply(m.1[,1,],1,sum)
```

We use the R function apply to compute the sum of the columns of the matrices cost.0 and cost.1 in the two columns of the matrix c. Similarly, we compute the total number of weeks in the state STW for each treatment in the matrix e. We are now ready to launch bcea to run the economic analysis.

```
labels <- c("FP","SFC")
m <- bcea(e,c,ref=2,interventions=labels,Kmax=300)
```

Notice that in this case it is useful to consider a very small value for the option Kmax. This is due to the fact that the two interventions are associated with similar costs, while the effectiveness of the new intervention is relatively large, thus generating a small ICER. Of course, this finding is generally not known before running the cost-effectiveness analysis.

Figure 5.12 shows a graphical summary of the results of the cost-effectiveness analysis. As suggested above, the ICER is exceptionally small (only £9). Consequently, $t = 1$ results in the optimal intervention for virtually any willingness-to-pay threshold.

Uncertainty about this result is also quite limited: the CEAC reaches values of 0.8 for $k \approx £50$, while the EVPI is at most £40 per patient, a very small amount.

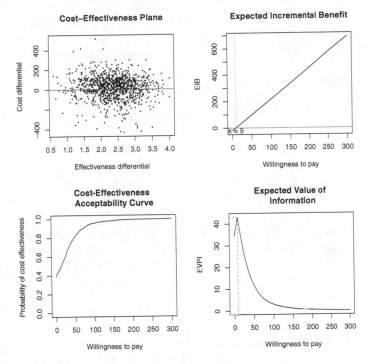

FIGURE 5.12
Summary of the health economic evaluation for the asthma model.

It is worth mentioning the relative sensitivity of the results to the scale of Dirichlet prior distributions. For example, if we set $\alpha_s^{(t)} = 0.5$ for all s, then ICER = £18. On the contrary, if $\alpha_s^{(t)} = 10$ for all s, then ICER = 0 and the uncertainty on the cost-effectiveness of $t = 1$ is virtually non-existent, with CEAC= 0.8 for $k = 0$ and EVPI $\approx$ £10 for k as small as £50.

In this case, however, despite the fact that the results are affected by the parametric assumptions used, it is important to remark that the final decision is not, and $t = 1$ can be considered as a cost-effective intervention with only limited uncertainty attached to this evaluation.

5.4.5 Adding memory to Markov models

The Markov property which characterises an MM implies that the future transitions of the patients do not depend on the complete history that has led them to sojourn in a particular state at a given time point, but only on the previous step. While this assumption has the effect of simplifying some of the calculations involved in running the MM, it may also represent a limitation.

Consider for instance the fictional example depicted in Figure 5.13. In this case, individuals can only be healthy, or diagnosed with cancer, or dead. Over time, it is possible to remain healthy, or to go through several periods in the disease stage and therefore both In health and Cancer are recurrent (or *transient*) states. In this simple example, we also assume that cancer patients can revert to the healthy state.

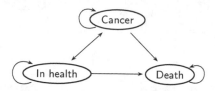

FIGURE 5.13

A hypothetical MM to describe the natural history of cancer patients. Individuals can only be healthy, or diagnosed with cancer, or dead. Both In health and Cancer are recurrent states and from both the patients can move to the absorbing state Death. Cancer patients can also be cured and return to the state In health.

Under the MM structure of Figure 5.13, we generally assume a probability λ_{j23} describing the transition between Cancer (indicated as $s = 2$) and Death ($s' = 3$) from time $(j-1)$ to time j. This implies that as time passes, mortality for cancer can change. For instance, if we simulate a virtual follow-up for a cohort of patients aged a at time j, it is reasonable to assume that mortality will be higher at time $(j+l)$, with $l > 0$, than it was at time j, simply because of the underlying ageing process.

Nevertheless, because of the Markov property, this model fails to account for the fact that, presumably, mortality from cancer is affected by the time spent in this state. In fact it is reasonable to assume that if a cancer patient survives the first few years (for the sake of simplicity, we consider in this example a period of three years), generally their cancer-related mortality becomes lower and eventually after a long enough period they can be considered cured from the disease and revert to the healthy state.

One possible solution is to consider a set of *tunnel* states, that can be used to keep track of the time spent in a given condition, effectively "adding memory" to the Markov structure. For example, the MM for the cancer problem can be modified to the one represented in Figure 5.14.

While the nodes In health and Death are unchanged, sojourns in the state of Cancer are now broken down into three time periods. More importantly, we can define different probabilities of death from each of the cancer stages, for example $\lambda_{25} \geq \lambda_{35} \geq \lambda_{45}$, where $s = 2, 3, 4$ indicate the three cancer stages and $s' = 5$ indicates death (these may of course depend on the time j). By considering a more complex structure, these transition probabilities account for the time spent with cancer, effectively overcoming the problem of the

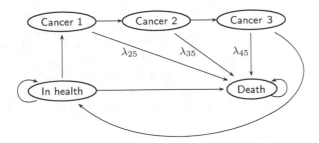

FIGURE 5.14
A hypothetical MM to describe the natural history of cancer patients by means of tunnel nodes. New cancer patients have a probability of death of λ_{25}, which is different (and in general greater) than that of patients who have had cancer for one period (λ_{35}). Similarly, patients who have had cancer for two time periods have yet a different probability of death λ_{45}, which is typically even lower. If a patient is not dead after three periods with cancer, they are assumed to go back to the state of health, from which they can re-enter the cancer loop.

absence of memory beyond the state in which the patients were in the previous time point.

The obvious limitation of the use of tunnel states is that the overall structure of the MM can become quite complicated; the increased number of nodes can also pose problems from the computational point of view. Nevertheless, this strategy is particularly effective in extending the applicability of MM to situations where the Markov property does not hold (at least for some of the states).

5.4.6 Indirect estimation of the transition probabilities

As mentioned earlier, it is not always possible to find direct evidence to estimate the relevant transition probabilities for a MM. For example, there can be no study evaluating the chance that patients move from one particular clinical state to another. In these cases, in order to use the machinery of the MM we need to estimate the transition probabilities using more complex methods.

Often, it is possible to link the transition probability from state s to state s' in two consecutive time points ($j-1$) and j to some relevant parameters. In other words we can define $\lambda_{jss'}$ as a deterministic function of some random quantities. Often, this kind of analysis is performed using simple models where these quantities are inputed using point estimations, e.g. in a spreadsheet. The full uncertainty in the underlying parameters is then not completely characterised, although sometimes MC analysis or DSA are also performed.

In a full Bayesian approach, the main parameters can be estimated using the available evidence, perhaps through a synthesis of the available literature as in §5.3. Thus, the resulting transition probabilities are computed as functions of random quantities, which induces a full posterior distribution accounting for the uncertainty in the economic model. As usual, this automatically produces a framework for PSA that is particularly straightforward to run, once the Bayesian model has been put in place.

To give an example, we consider here a simplified version of the MM presented in Cooper et al. (2004). The structure of the problem is presented in Figure 5.15. The relevant population is represented by patients with metastatic breast cancer and surviving an initial cycle of treatment with two different chemotherapy drugs. Doxorubicin ($t = 0$) is the drug currently used, while Docetaxel ($t = 1$) is the treatment whose cost-effectiveness is being assessed.

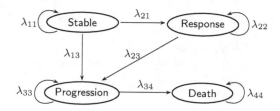

FIGURE 5.15

The simplified version of the MM for the metastatic breast cancer. Source Cooper et al. (2004).

The MM assumes three-week cycles to coincide with the chemotherapy treatment intervals. Patients who have survived up to this point can sojourn in one of the following states: **Stable** indicates no change in the disease state; **Response** indicates complete or partial tumor disappearance; **Progression** identifies tumour growth or spread; and **Death**.

As suggested earlier, no direct evidence exists to estimate the required transition probabilities. However, we can combine information available from alternative sources of evidence (such as RCTs) and then define the transition probabilities as logical functions of suitably defined random quantities. In particular, we consider the following sub-models.

Sub-model 1. Evidence synthesis model for the probability of response

The first set of available data consists of results from $N_0^{\text{res}} = 2$ and $N_1^{\text{res}} = 4$ RCTs investigating the response of patients for $t = 0$ and 1 respectively. In each study $i = 1, \ldots, N_t^{\text{res}}$ and for each intervention $t = (0, 1)$, the observed variable is the number of patients who have a response, which we indicate with r_{ti}^{res}, out of the n_{ti}^{res} observed.

We model the data using the formulation below

$$r_{ti}^{\text{res}} \sim \text{Binomial}(p_{ti}^{\text{res}}, n_{ti}^{\text{res}})$$
$$\text{logit}(p_{ti}^{\text{res}}) = \delta_{ti}^{\text{res}} \sim \text{Normal}(\mu_t^{\text{res}}, \sigma_t^{\text{res}})$$
$$\mu_t^{\text{res}} \sim \text{Normal}(0, v^{\text{res}}) \quad \text{and} \quad \sigma_t^{\text{res}} \sim \text{Uniform}(0, w^{\text{res}})$$
$$\pi_t^{\text{res}} = \frac{\exp(\mu_t^{\text{res}})}{1 + \exp(\mu_t^{\text{res}})},$$

for some large constant v^{res} and w^{res}. Here, the parameters p_{ti}^{res} are the study- and treatment-specific probability of response, while the variable μ_t^{res} represents the pooled probability of response and σ_t^{res} is the standard deviation. Both these quantities are defined on the logit scale; thus the parameter π_t^{res} is then computed to rescale this quantity on the natural $[0; 1]$ scale. Notice that π_t^{res} does not directly represent one of the relevant transition probabilities. However, as we will show later, it can be used to derive them using suitable deterministic relationships.

Sub-model 2. Evidence synthesis model for the probability of toxicity

The second set of data informs about the chance of discontinuation of treatment due to toxicity. In particular, there are $N_0^{\text{tox}} = 2$ and $N_1^{\text{tox}} = 3$ studies for $t = 0$ and 1 respectively, in which, similarly to the previous case, the records are the number r_{ti}^{tox} of patients who discontinue treatment out of the n_{ti}^{tox} observed. We use the same formulation as in the model above

$$r_{ti}^{\text{tox}} \sim \text{Binomial}(p_{ti}^{\text{tox}}, n_{ti}^{\text{tox}})$$
$$\text{logit}(p_{ti}^{\text{tox}}) = \delta_{ti}^{\text{tox}} \sim \text{Normal}(\mu_t^{\text{tox}}, \sigma_t^{\text{tox}})$$
$$\mu_t^{\text{tox}} \sim \text{Normal}(0, v^{\text{tox}}) \quad \text{and} \quad \sigma_t^{\text{tox}} \sim \text{Uniform}(0, w^{\text{tox}})$$
$$\pi_t^{\text{tox}} = \frac{\exp(\mu_t^{\text{tox}})}{1 + \exp(\mu_t^{\text{tox}})},$$

so that the pooled probability of toxicity is obtained and computed as π_t^{tox}.

Sub-model 3. Model for the time to response

The next module considers data derived by one RCT in which the two treatments have been compared in terms of the median time to response, x_t^{tr}. As is often the case with this type of outcome variable, the available data are represented by some observed summary (usually, the median) of the time to the event of interest and some measure of the observed (or estimated) variability, such as the variance ϕ_t^{tr}, which in this case we consider as a known quantity.

The availability of this kind of data is not directly relevant to the construction of the MM, but using some simplifying assumptions about the underlying survival process and the observed data, it is possible to rescale the median time to the event in terms of a probability parameter, which can then be used to construct the required transition probabilities.

Given that the median time to response is a continuous variable, at least as a first approximation we can model it as

$$x_t^{\text{tr}} \sim \text{Normal}(\mu_t^{\text{tr}}, \phi_t^{\text{tr}})$$
$$\mu_t^{\text{tr}} \sim \text{Normal}(0, v^{\text{tr}})\mathbb{I}(0, \infty)$$

where μ_t^{tr} represents the average of the distribution of the median time to event and v^{tr} is a large constant (of course prior knowledge of the median time could be encoded by assuming more informative structures for v^{tr}. Similarly, additional covariates could be included in a more complex specification of the model).

Notice that because both x_t^{tr} and μ_t^{tr} are by definition positive quantities, the Normal models used here may not be the most appropriate, in general. One possibility, which we consider here, is to truncate these distributions, constraining them to assume only values in $[0, \infty)$. This is particularly relevant for the unobserved parameter μ_t^{tr} to which truncation is applied; because there is direct evidence, this may be less of a problem for x_t^{tr}, but alternative, more complex models (e.g. logNormal or Gamma) probably could be used instead. Despite using a slightly different notation, both JAGS and BUGS allow the user to specify truncated distributions (cfr. the software manuals and help files).

Second, if we assume that the time to response has an Exponential distribution, for each treatment t the survival curve at time j (expressing the proportion of subjects who have not yet experienced the event under study) is

$$S_t^{\text{tr}}(j) = \exp\left(-\rho_t^{\text{tr}} j\right), \tag{5.13}$$

where ρ_t^{tr} is a *constant hazard*, i.e. the instant probability of moving from the state Stable to the state Response under treatment t. At any time point j, this can be estimated as

$$\rho_t^{\text{tr}} = -\frac{\log\left(S_t^{\text{tr}}(j)\right)}{j} \tag{5.14}$$

by taking the logarithm of both sides and simply re-arranging (5.13). In particular, if we evaluate (5.14) at the median time (which can be estimated by its mean μ_t^{tr}), it is easy to derive that

$$\rho_t^{\text{tr}} = -\frac{\log(0.5)}{\mu_t^{\text{tr}}},$$

since, by definition, the proportion of survivors at the median time is 0.5.

Finally, because the cycles of the MM are defined in terms of three-week periods, it is necessary to rescale the hazard accordingly in order to compute the cycle-specific probability of moving from Stable to Response using the generic relationship (Miller and Homan, 1994; Cooper et al., 2004)

$$\beta_t^{\text{tr}} = 1 - \exp\left(-\frac{\rho_t^{\text{tr}}}{\tau}\right),$$

where τ is the length of the MM cycles (e.g. 3 weeks in this case).

Sub-model 4. Evidence synthesis model for the time to progression

The fourth sub-model consists of data about the median time to progression. Again, these are not directly usable to compute a transition probability, but can be manipulated to produce the required estimation indirectly.

In this case, there are $N_0^{\text{tp}} = 2$ and $N_1^{\text{tp}} = 4$ studies reporting the median time to reach the state of progression, which we indicate as x_{ti}^{tp} for treatment t and study i, together with an estimation of the variability associated with this quantity, which we indicate as ϕ_{ti}^{tp} and again consider as a known constant.

Because in this case there are a few studies investigating the same quantity, it is possible to produce a pooled estimation, by means of a suitable hierarchical model that allows us to combine the observations deriving from the different sources. We do so by modelling the average median time to progression δ_{ti}^{tp} using an exchangeable formulation.

$$x_{ti}^{\text{tp}} \sim \text{Normal}(\delta_{ti}^{\text{tp}}, \phi_{ti}^{\text{tp}})$$
$$\delta_{ti}^{\text{tp}} \sim \text{Normal}(\mu_t^{\text{tp}}, \sigma_t^{\text{tp}})$$
$$\mu_t^{\text{tp}} \sim \text{Normal}(0, v^{\text{tp}})\mathbb{I}(0, \infty) \quad \text{and} \quad \sigma_t^{\text{tp}} \sim \text{Uniform}(0, w^{\text{tp}})$$

In the above formulation, μ_t^{tp} and σ_t^{tp} represent the pooled average and standard deviation for the median time for each treatment t. For simplicity, the quantities v^{tp} and w^{tp} are again assumed as large constant values.

The three-week specific probability of moving to progression can be estimated by means of the same reasoning used above

$$\rho_t^{\text{tp}} = \frac{-\log(0.5)}{\mu_t^{\text{tp}}}$$
$$\beta_t^{\text{tp}} = 1 - \exp(-\rho_t^{\text{tp}}/3).$$

The quantity β_t^{tp} will be used to characterise the relevant transition probability to be applied in the MM.

Sub-model 5. Evidence synthesis model for survival time

The last source of information available concerns the median survival time. This is estimated using data from $N_0^{\text{srv}} = 2$ and $N_1^{\text{srv}} = 3$ studies in which the two treatment under consideration have been analysed. We follow the same specification as for two previous sub-models, in order to estimate the average median survival time μ_t^{srv}.

$$x_{ti}^{\text{srv}} \sim \text{Normal}(\delta_{ti}^{\text{srv}}, \phi_{ti}^{\text{srv}})$$
$$\delta_{ti}^{\text{srv}} \sim \text{Normal}(\mu_t^{\text{srv}}, \sigma_t^{\text{srv}})$$
$$\mu_t^{\text{srv}} \sim \text{Normal}(0, v^{\text{srv}})\mathbb{I}(0, \infty) \quad \text{and} \quad \sigma_t^{\text{srv}} \sim \text{Uniform}(0, w^{\text{srv}})$$

Notice that this parameter is not directly of interest but will again be used to construct a functional relationship that will allow us to estimate a further parameter that in turn will be used to determine one of the required transition probabilities.

Sub-model 6. Model for the time to death

The final sub-model allows us to estimate the time from progression to death. There are no directly relevant data on this transition; however, we can use the results of the previous two sub-models to estimate the corresponding three-week probability by means of the following specification.

First, we note that because transitions towards the state Death only occur from the state Progression, the difference between the median survival time and the median time to progression represents an estimation of the time that a random patient treated with t spends in the state of Progression before moving to Death.

Therefore, even without direct data it is possible to estimate the average of the median time from progression to death as

$$\mu_t^{\mathrm{dth}} = \mu_t^{\mathrm{srv}} - \mu_t^{\mathrm{tp}}.$$

Notice that within the Bayesian approach and for instance using MCMC procedures, a sample from the posterior distributions of both μ_t^{srv} and μ_t^{tp} will be available. Thus, combining them, a sample from the posterior distribution of μ_t^{dth} will be automatically induced.

Then, using the same reasoning discussed above, we can estimate the three-week probability of moving from Progression to Death as

$$\rho_t^{\mathrm{dth}} = \frac{-\log(0.5)}{\mu_t^{\mathrm{dth}}}$$

$$\beta_t^{\mathrm{dth}} = 1 - \exp(-\rho_t^{\mathrm{dth}}/3).$$

Computing the transition probabilities

We can now compute the transition probabilities for the MM of Figure 5.15 as logical functions of the vector of parameters $\boldsymbol{\theta} = (\pi_t^{\mathrm{res}}, \pi_t^{\mathrm{tox}}, \beta_t^{\mathrm{tr}}, \beta_t^{\mathrm{dth}})$. First, we consider the transitions off the state Stable. If a patient experiences toxicity, which happens with probability π_t^{tox}, then they will move towards the state Progression. Thus, it is straightforward to model $\lambda_{13}^{(t)} = \pi_t^{\mathrm{tox}}$.

On the other hand, patients who do not experience toxicity, which obviously happens with probability $(1 - \pi_t^{\mathrm{tox}})$ can either remain stable or move towards the state Response. Using the results of the models described above, the latter occurs with probability β_t^{tr}. Thus, we can model $\lambda_{12}^{(t)} = (1 - \pi_t^{\mathrm{tox}})\beta_t^{\mathrm{tr}}$. Obviously, the probability of remaining in the state Stable is then computed as $\lambda_{11}^{(t)} = (1 - \pi_t^{\mathrm{tox}})(1 - \beta_t^{\mathrm{tr}})$.

Notice that in this case it is straightforward to check that

$$
\begin{aligned}
\sum_{s'=1}^{S} \lambda_{1s'}^{(t)} &= \lambda_{11}^{(t)} + \lambda_{12}^{(t)} + \lambda_{13}^{(t)} \\
&= [(1 - \pi_t^{\text{tox}})(1 - \beta_t^{\text{tr}})] + [(1 - \pi_t^{\text{tox}})\beta_t^{\text{tr}}] + [\pi_t^{\text{tox}}] \\
&= 1,
\end{aligned}
$$

i.e. the transitions out of the state Stable sum to 1. In fact, because this condition needs to always hold, it would be sufficient to compute all but one of the required transition probabilities and derive the remaining one setting it at 1 minus the sum of all the others.

Using a similar reasoning, consider a patient who is in the state Response and does not experience toxicity. If they have a positive response, which happens with probability π_t^{res}, then they will remain in that state and thus we can set $\lambda_{22}^{(t)} = (1 - \pi_t^{\text{tox}})\pi_t^{\text{res}}$. On the other hand, there are two possible situations which will see them move to the state Progression. This can happen (a) directly, if they experience toxicity; or (b) indirectly, if they do not experience toxicity but they do not have a response.

Because cases (a) and (b) are mutually exclusive (i.e. they cannot happen at the same time), we can apply the law of total probability and model $\lambda_{23}^{(t)} = \pi_t^{\text{tox}} + (1 - \pi_t^{\text{tox}})(1 - \pi_t^{\text{res}})$. Again, we can see that the sum of the admissible transitions out of the state Response sums to 1, as required.

As for the transitions out of the state Progression, it is easy to see that the probability of moving to death is simply estimated as $\lambda_{34}^{(t)} = \beta_t^{\text{dth}}$ and thus we can set the probability of remaining in this state as $\lambda_{33}^{(t)} = 1 - \beta_t^{\text{dth}}$.

Finally, since Death is, as usual, an absorbent state, we have that $\lambda_{44}^{(t)} = 1$ and $\lambda_{4s'}^{(t)} = 0$ for all $s' \neq 4$.

JAGS implementation

We code the model described above using the following specification

```
model {
  # Sub-model 1
    for (i in 1:N.res[1]) {
        r.res1[i] ~ dbin(p.res1[i],n.res1[i])
        logit(p.res1[i]) <- delta.res1[i]
        delta.res1[i] ~ dnorm(mu.res[1],tau.res[1])
  }
    for (i in 1:N.res[2]) {
        r.res2[i] ~ dbin(p.res2[i],n.res2[i])
        logit(p.res2[i]) <- delta.res2[i]
        delta.res2[i] ~ dnorm(mu.res[2],tau.res[2])
  }
```

```
    for (t in 1:2) {
        mu.res[t] ~ dnorm(0,prec.mu.res)
        sigma.res[t] ~ dunif(0,w.res)
        tau.res[t] <- pow(sigma.res[t],-2)
        pi.res[t] <- exp(mu.res[t])/(1+exp(mu.res[t]))
    }

  # Sub-model 2
    for (i in 1:N.tox[1]) {
        r.tox1[i] ~ dbin(p.tox1[i],n.tox1[i])
        logit(p.tox1[i]) <- delta.tox1[i]
        delta.tox1[i] ~ dnorm(mu.tox[1],tau.tox[1])
    }
    for (i in 1:N.tox[2]) {
        r.tox2[i] ~ dbin(p.tox2[i],n.tox2[i])
        logit(p.tox2[i]) <- delta.tox2[i]
        delta.tox2[i] ~ dnorm(mu.tox[2],tau.tox[2])
    }
    for (t in 1:2) {
        mu.tox[t] ~ dnorm(0,prec.mu.tox)
        sigma.tox[t] ~ dunif(0,w.tox)
        tau.tox[t] <- pow(sigma.tox[t],-2)
        pi.tox[t] <- exp(mu.tox[t])/(1+exp(mu.tox[t]))
    }

  # Sub-model 3
    for (t in 1:2) {
        x.tr[t] ~ dnorm(mu.tr[t],prec.tr[t])
        mu.tr[t] ~ dnorm(0,prec.tr)T(0,)
        rho.tr[t] <- -log(0.5)/mu.tr[t]
        beta.tr[t] <- 1-exp(-rho.tr[t]/tau)
        prec.tr[t] <- 1/phi.tr[t]
    }

  # Sub-model 4
    for (i in 1:N.tp[1]) {
        x.tp1[i] ~ dnorm(delta.tp1[i],prec.tp1[i])
        delta.tp1[i] ~ dnorm(mu.tp[1],tau.tp[1])
        prec.tp1[i] <- 1/phi.tp1[i]
    }
    for (i in 1:N.tp[2]) {
        x.tp2[i] ~ dnorm(delta.tp2[i],prec.tp2[i])
        delta.tp2[i] ~ dnorm(mu.tp[2],tau.tp[2])
        prec.tp2[i] <- 1/phi.tp2[i]
    }
```

```
    for (t in 1:2) {
        mu.tp[t] ~ dnorm(0,prec.mu.tp[t])T(0,)
        sigma.tp[t] ~ dunif(0,w.tp)
        prec.mu.tp[t] <- pow(sigma.tp[t],-2)
        rho.tp[t] <- -log(0.5)/mu.tp[t]
        beta.tp[t] <- 1-exp(-rho.tp[t]/tau)
    }

# Sub-model 5
    for (i in 1:N.srv[1]) {
        x.srv1[i] ~ dnorm(delta.srv1[i],prec.srv1[i])
        delta.srv1[i] ~ dnorm(mu.srv[1],tau.srv[1])
        prec.srv1[i] <- 1/phi.srv1[i]
    }
    for (i in 1:N.srv[2]) {
        x.srv2[i] ~ dnorm(delta.srv2[i],prec.srv2[i])
        delta.srv2[i] ~ dnorm(mu.srv[2],tau.srv[2])
        prec.srv2[i] <- 1/phi.srv2[i]
    }
    for (t in 1:2) {
        mu.srv[t] ~ dnorm(0,prec.mu.srv[t])T(0,)
        sigma.srv[t] ~ dunif(0,w.srv)
        prec.mu.srv[t] <- pow(sigma.srv[t],-2)
        rho.srv[t] <- -log(0.5)/mu.srv[t]
        beta.srv[t] <- 1-exp(-rho.srv[t]/tau)
    }

# Sub-model 6
    for (t in 1:2) {
        mu.dth[t] <- mu.srv[t] - mu.tp[t]
        rho.dth[t] <- -log(0.5)/mu.dth[t]
        beta.dth[t] <- 1-exp(-rho.dth[t]/tau)
    }
}
```

Notice that JAGS codes truncated distributions using the notation $T(\cdot,\cdot)$, while BUGS uses the slightly different notation $I(\cdot,\cdot)$. In either case, the extremes of the truncation interval are specified inside the brackets. In the present code, in order to force the distribution of the averages of the median times to be positive, we use the notation $T(0,)$.

The relevant data can be loaded in R using the following code.

```
# Data on the probability of response (sub-model 1)
N.res <- c(2,4)              # Number of studies
r.res0 <- c(55,42)           # Cases for t=0
n.res0 <- c(165,118)         # Total observations for t=0
r.res1 <- c(77,61,61,25)     # Cases for t=1
```

```
n.res1 <- c(161,203,143,46)     # Total observations for t=1

# Data on the probability of toxicity (sub-model 2)
N.tox <- c(2,4)                     # Number of studies
r.tox0 <- c(55,42)                  # Cases for t=0
n.tox0 <- c(165,118)                # Total observations for t=0
r.tox1 <- c(77,61,61,25)            # Cases for t=1
n.tox1 <- c(161,203,143,46)         # Total observations for t=1

# Data on time to response (sub-model 3)
x.tr <- c(23,12)                    # Observed median time
phi.tr <- c(3,3)^2                  # Observed variance
prec.tr <- 1/phi.tr                 # Computed precision

# Data on time to progression (sub-model 4)
N.tp <- c(2,3)                          # Number of studies
x.tp1 <- c(23,21)                       # Observed median time (t=0)
phi.tp1 <- c(4.077,1.943)^2             # Observed variance (t=0)
prec.tp1 <- 1/phi.tp1                   # Computed precision (t=0)
x.tp2 <- c(19,26,27.3)                  # Observed median time (t=1)
phi.tp2 <- c(2.048,2.263,1.631)^2 # Observed variance (t=1)
prec.tp2 <- 1/phi.tp2                   # Computed precision (t=1)
tau <- 3                                # MM cycle length

# Data on survival time (sub-model 5)
N.srv <- c(2,3)                         # Number of studies
x.srv1 <- c(60.66,47)                   # Observed median time (t=0)
phi.srv1 <- c(3.9723,5.6880)^2          # Observed variance (t=0)
prec.srv1 <- 1/phi.srv1                 # Computed precision (t=0)
x.srv2 <- c(47.67,65,45.07)             # Observed median time (t=1)
phi.srv2 <- c(4.845,5.171,2.174)^2 # Observed variance (t=1)
prec.srv2 <- 1/phi.srv2                 # Computed precision (t=1)
```

The model can be run in JAGS, to produce an estimation of the relevant parameters, which can in turn be used to generate the MM exactly as specified in §5.4.4, i.e. by defining the virtual cohort and simulating the virtual follow-up.

Cost-effectiveness analysis

For each time $j = 1, \ldots, J$ and for each state, it is possible to record the associated costs and measure of effectiveness, which can be discounted, if suitable, using the general formulation shown earlier.

Of course, both costs and benefits can be defined in an additional sub-model, for instance using a suitable specification based on available data or expert opinions to account for the underlying uncertainty. This step, however, does not imply any extra difficulty with respect to the models shown in the previous sections.

The simulations obtained from the MM can be used to define the suitable variables of cost and effect in the population that are then used as inputs to the function bcea, which performs the actual economic analysis. In particular we note again here that under the Bayesian approach based on MCMC simulations, because all the random quantites are estimated by means of draws from the posterior distributions, any logical function defined starting from them will also be associated with a vector, matrix, or array of values from its posterior distribution.

References

Ades, A., K. Claxton, and M. Sculpher (2006). Evidence synthesis, parameter correlation and probabilistic sensitivity analysis. *Health Economics 15*, 373–381.

Ades, A., G. Lu, and K. Claxton (2004). Expected value of sample information calculations in medical decision modeling. *Medical Decision-Making 24*, 207–227.

Ades, A. and A. Sutton (2006). Multiparameter evidence synthesis in epidemiology and medical decision-making: Current approaches. *Journal of the Royal Statistical Society* A *169*, 5–35.

Albert, J. (2007). *Bayesian Computation with R*. Springer-Verlag, New York, NY.

Arbuthnot, J. (1710). An argument for Divine Providence, taken from the constant regularity observed in the births of both sexes. *Philosophical Transactions of the Royal Society of London 27*, 186–190.

Baio, G. (2012). BCEA: A package to run Bayesian Cost-Effectiveness Analysis in R. https://sites.google.com/a/statistica.it/gianluca/bcea.

Baio, G. and P. Dawid (2011). Probabilistic sensitivity analysis in health economics. *Statistical Methods in Medical Research doi: 0962280211419832*, First published 18 September 2011.

Baio, G. and P. Russo (2009). A decision-theoretic framework for the application of cost-effectiveness analysis in regulatory processes. *Pharmacoeconomics 27 (8)*, 645–655.

Barber, J. and S. Thompson (1998). Analysis and interpretation of cost data in randomised controlled trials: Review of published studies. *British Medical Journal 317*, 1195–1200.

Bayes, T. (1763). Essay towards solving a problem in the doctrine of chances. *Philosophical Transactions of the Royal Society of London 53*, 370–418.

Bennet, K., G. Torrence, M. Boyle, and R. Guscot (2000). Cost-utility analysis in depression: The McSad utility measure for depression health states. *Psychiatric Services 51(9)*, 1171–1176.

Berger, J. (1985). *Statistical Decision Theory and Bayesian Analysis, 2nd edition*. Springer-Verlag, New York, NY.

Bernardo, J. and A. Smith (1999). *Bayesian Theory*. John Wiley & Sons, New York, NY.

Berry, D. (1996). *Statistics: A Bayesian Perspective*. Duxbury, London, UK.

Bertsch McGrayne, S. (2011). *The Theory That Would Not Die: How Bayes' Rule Cracked the Enigma Code, Hunted Down Russian Submarines, and Emerged Triumphant from Two Centuries of Controversy*. Yale University Press, New Haven, CT.

Berwick, D. (2005). Broadening the view of evidence-based medicine. *International Journal of Quality and Safety in Health Care 14*, 315–316.

Brazier, J. (2010). Is the EQ-5D fit for purpose in mental health? *British Journal of Psychiatry 197*, 348–349.

Brazier, J., J. Ratcliffe, A. Tsuchiya, and J. Salomon (2007a). *Measuring and Valuing Health Benefits for Economic Evaluations*. Oxford University Press, Oxford, UK.

Brazier, J., J. Roberts, and M. Deverill (2002). The estimation of a preference-based measure of health from the SF-36. *Journal of Health Economics 21(2)*, 271–292.

Brazier, J., J. Roberts, A. Tsuchiya, and J. Busschbach (2004). A comparison of the EQ-5D and the SF-6D across seven patient groups. *Health Economics 13*, 873–884.

Brazier, J., Y. Yang, and A. Tsuchiya (2007b). *Review of Methods for Mapping between Condition Specific Measures onto Generic Measures of Health*. Office of Health Economics, London, UK.

Brennan, A. and S. Kharroubi (2005). Efficient Computation of Partial Expected Value of Sample Information Using Bayesian Approximation. Research Report 560/05, Department of Probability and Statistics, University of Sheffield, UK.

Brennan, A., S. Kharroubi, A. O'Hagan, and J. Chilcott (2007). Calculating partial expected value of perfect information via Monte Carlo sampling algorithms. *Medical Decision-Making 27*, 448–470.

Briggs, A. (2000). Handling uncertainty in cost-effectiveness models. *Pharmacoeconomics 22*, 479–500.

Briggs, A., A. Ades, and M. Price (2003). Probabilistic sensitivity analysis for decision trees with multiple branches: Use of the Dirichlet distribution in a Bayesian framework. *Medical Decision-Making 23*, 341–350.

Briggs, A., R. Goeree, G. Blackhouse, and B. O' Brien (2002). Probabilistic analysis of cost-effectiveness models: Choosing between treatment strategies for gastroesophageal reflux disease. *Medical Decision-Making 4*, 290–308.

Briggs, A. and A. Gray (1998). The distribution of health care costs and their statistical analysis for economic evaluation. *Journal of Health Services Research and Policy 3*, 233–245.

Briggs, A. and B. O' Brien (2001). The death of cost-minimisation analysis? *Journal of Health Economics 10*, 179–184.

Briggs, A. and M. Sculpher (1998). Introducing Markov models for economic evaluation. *Pharmacoeconomics 13(4)*, 397–409.

Briggs, A., M. Sculpher, and K. Claxton (2006). *Decision Modelling for Health Economic Evaluation*. Oxford University Press, Oxford, UK.

Brooks, S., A. Gelman, G. Jones, and X. Meng (2011). *Handbook of Markov Chain Monte Carlo*. Chapman & Hall/CRC, Boca Raton, FL.

Brouwer, W., L. Niessen, M. Postma, and F. Rutten (2005). Need for differential discounting of costs and health effects in cost-effectiveness analyses. *British Medical Journal 331(7514)*, 446 448.

Browne, W. and D. Draper (2006). A comparison of Bayesian and likelihood-based methods for fitting multilevel models. *Bayesian Analysis 1(3)*, 473–517.

Carlin, B. and T. Louis (2009). *Bayesian methods for data analysis 3rd edition*. Chapman & Hall/CRC, Boca Raton, FL.

Christensen, R., W. Johnson, A. Branscum, and T. Hanson (2011). *Bayesian Ideas and Data Analyses*. Chapman & Hall/CRC, Boca Raton, FL.

Claxton, K. (1999a). Bayesian approaches to the value of information: Implications for the regulation of new pharmaceutical. *Health Economics 8*, 269–274.

Claxton, K. (1999b). The irrelevance of inference: A decision-making approach to stochastic evaluation of health care technologies. *Journal of Health Economics 18*, 342–364.

Claxton, K., L. Lacey, and S. Walker (2000). Selecting treatments: A decision theoretic approach. *Journal of the Royal Statistical Society A 163*, 211–225.

Claxton, K., P. Neumann, S. Araki, and M. Weinstein (2001). Bayesian value-of-information analysis. *International Journal of Technology Assessment in Health Care 17*, 38–55.

Claxton, K., M. Sculpher, C. McCabe, A. Briggs, R. Akehurst, M. Buxton, J. Brazier, and A. O'Hagan (2005). Probabilistic sensitivity analysis for NICE technology assessment: Not an optional extra. *Health Economics 14*, 339–347.

Congdon, P. (2001). *Bayesian Statistical Modelling*. John Wiley & Sons, Chichester, UK.

Congdon, P. (2003). *Applied Bayesian Modelling*. John Wiley & Sons, Chichester, UK.

Congdon, P. (2010). *Applied Bayesian Hierarchical Methods*. CRC Press, Boca Raton, FL.

Conigliani, C. and A. Tancredi (2009). A Bayesian model averaging approach for cost-effectiveness analysis. *Health Economics 18(7)*, 807–821.

Cooper, N., P. Lambert, K. Abrams, and A. Sutton (2007). Predicting costs over time using Bayesian Markov Chain Monte Carlo methods: An application to early inflammatory polyarthritis. *Health Economics 16*, 37–56.

Cooper, N., A. Sutton, K. Abrams, D. Turner, and A. Wailoo (2004). Comprehensive decision analytical modelling in economic evaluation: A Bayesian approach. *Health Economics 13(3)*, 203–226.

Cooper, N., A. Sutton, M. Mugford, and K. Abrams (2003). Use of Bayesian Markov Chain Monte Carlo methods to model cost-of-illness data. *Medical Decision-Making*, 23–38.

Coyle, D. and J. Oakley (2008). Estimating the expected value of partial perfect information: A review of methods. *European Journal of Health Economics 9*, 251–259.

Dawid, P. (1979). Conditional independence in statistical theory (with discussion). *Journal of the Royal Statistical Society, B 41*, 1–31.

Dawid, P. (2005). Probability and Proof. In T. Anderson, D. Schum, and W. Twining (Eds.), *Analysis of Evidence – 2nd Edition*. Cambridge University Press, Cambridge, UK.

Dawson, J., H. Doll, C. Jenkinson, and A. Carr (2010). The routine use of patient reported outcome measures in healthcare settings. *British Medical Journal 340*, 464–467.

de Finetti, B. (1974). *Theory of Probability*, Volume 1. John Wiley & Sons, New York, NY.

Department of Health of the Commonwealth of Australia (1992). *Guidelines for the Pharmaceutical Industry on Preparation of Submissions to the Pharmaceutical Benefits Advisory Committee, Including Submissions Involving*

Economic Analyses. Australian Government Publishing Service, Canberra, Australia.

Devlin, N., A. Tsuchiya, K. Buckingham, and C. Tilling (2011). A uniform time trade off method for states better and worse than dead: Feasibility study of the 'lead time' approach. *Health Economics 20(3)*, 348–361.

Dolan, P., C. Gudex, P. Kind, and A. Williams (1995). *A Social Tariff for Euroqol: Results from a UK general population survey*. Centre for Health Economics, University of York, York, UK.

Donaldson, C. and K. Gerard (2005). *The Economics of Health Care Financing: The Visible Hand*. Palgrave MacMillan, New York, NY.

Doubilet, P., C. Begg, M. Weinstein, P. Braun, and B. McNeil (1985). Probabilistic sensitivity analysis using Monte Carlo simulation. A practical approach. *Medical Decision-Making 5*, 157–177.

Draper, D. (1995). Assessment and propagation of model uncertainty (with discussion). *Journal of the Royal Statistical Society, B 57*, 45–97.

Drummond, M., B. O'Brien, G. Stoddar, and G. Torrance (2005). *Methods for the Economic Evaluation of Health Care Programmes. Third Edition*. Oxford University Press, London, UK.

Eddy, D., V. Hasselblad, and R. Shachter (1990). A Bayesian method for synthesizing evidence: The confidence profile method. *International Journal of Technology Assessment in Health Care 6*, 31–55.

Edwards, D. (2000). *Introduction to Graphical Modelling 2nd edition*. Springer Verlag, New York, NY.

Felli, J. and G. Hazen (1998). Sensitivity analysis and the expected value of perfect information. *Medical Decision-Making 18*, 95–109.

Felli, J. and G. Hazen (1999). A Bayesian approach to sensitivity analysis. *Health Economics 8*, 263–268.

Fenwick, E., K. Claxton, and M. Sculpher (2001). Representing uncertainty: The role of cost effectiveness acceptability curves. *Health Economics 10*, 779–787.

Fenwick, E., B. O'Brien, and A. Briggs (2004). Cost-effectiveness acceptability curves — Facts, fallacies and frequently asked questions. *Health Economics 13*, 269–274.

Fenwick, E., S. Palmer, K. Claxton, M. Sculpher, K. Abrams, and A. Sutton (2006). An iterative Bayesian approach to health technology assessment: Application to a policy of preoperative optimization for patients undergoing major elective surgery. *Medical Decision-Making 26*, 480–496.

Fienberg, S. (2006). When did Bayesian inference become Bayesian? *Bayesian Analysis 1*, 1–40.

Folland, S., A. Goodman, and M. Stano (2012). *The Economics of Health and Health Care. Seventh Edition.* Prentice Hall, Upper Saddle River, NJ.

Gamerman, D. (1997). *Markov Chain Monte Carlo.* Chapman & Hall, London, UK.

Gelman, A. (2006). Prior distributions for variance parameters in hierarchical models. *Bayesian Analysis 1(3)*, 515–533.

Gelman, A., J. Carlin, H. Stern, and D. Rubin (2004). *Bayesian Data Analysis - 2nd edition.* Chapman & Hall, New York, NY.

Gelman, A. and J. Hill (2007). *Data Analysis Using Regression and Multi-level/Hierarchical Models.* Cambridge University Press, Cambridge, UK.

Gelman, A. and D. Rubin (1992). Inference from iterative simulation using multiple sequences. *Statistical Sciences 7*, 457–511.

Geman, S. and D. Geman (1984). Stochastic relaxation, Gibbs distributions, and the Bayesian restoration of images. *IEEE Transactions on Pattern Analysis and Machine Intelligence 6*, 721–741.

Gilks, W., S. Richardson, and D. Spiegelhalter (1996). *Markov Chain Monte Carlo in Practice.* Chapman & Hall, London, UK.

Gillies, D. (2000). *Philophical theories of probability.* Routledge, London, UK.

Girolami, M. and B. Calderhead (2011). Riemann manifold Langevin and Hamiltonian Monte Carlo methods. *Journal of the Royal Statistical Society B 73(2)*, 1–37.

Glick, A., J. Doshi, S. Sonnad, and D. Polsky (2007). *Economic Evaluation in Clinical Trials.* Oxford University Press, Oxford, UK.

Goodman, S. (1999). Toward evidence-based medical statistics. 1: The P value fallacy. *Annals of Internal Medicine 130*, 995–1004.

Griffin, S., K. Claxton, N. Hawkins, and M. Sculpher (2006). Probabilistic analysis and computationally expensive models: Necessary and required? *Value in Health 9*, 244–252.

Hastings, W. (1970). Monte Carlo sampling methods using Markov Chains and their applications. *Biometrika 57(1)*, 97–109.

Howard, R. (1966). Information value theory. *IEEE Transactions on System Science and Cybernetics*, (1) 22-26. SCC-2.

Howie, D. (2002). *Interpreting Probability*. Cambridge University Press, Cambridge, UK.

Hunnink, M. and P. Glasziou (2001). *Decision-making in Health and Medicine*. Cambridge University Press, Cambridge, UK.

Institute of Medicine (2008). *Improving the Quality of Cancer Clinical Trials: Workshop Summary*. The National Academies Press, Washington, DC.

Jackman, S. (2009). *Bayesian Analysis for the Social Sciences*. John Wiley & Sons, New York, NY.

Jackson, C., L. Boijke, S. Thompson, K. Claxton, and L. Sharples (2011). A framework for addressing structural uncertainty in decision models. *Medical Decision-Making 31*, 662–674.

Jackson, C., L. Sharples, and S. Thompson (2010). Structural and parameter uncertainty in Bayesian cost-effectiveness analysis. *Journal of the Royal Statistical Society, C 59*, 233–253.

Jackson, C., S. Thompson, and L. Sharples (2009). Accounting for uncertainty in health economic decision models by using model averaging. *Journal of the Royal Statistical Society, A 172(2)*, 383–404.

Jeffreys, H. (1961). *Theory of Probability*. Clarendon Press, Oxford, UK.

Jordaan, I. (2005). *Decisions under Uncertainty*. Cambridge University Press, Cambridge, UK.

Karroubi, S., J. Brazier, J. Roberts, and A. O'Hagan (2007). Modelling sf-6d health state preference data using a nonparametric Bayesian method. *Journal of Health Economics 26(3)*, 597–612.

Kind, P., R. Brooks, and R. Rabin (2005). *EQ-5D Concepts and Methods: A Developmental History*. Springer, Dordrecht, The Netherlands.

King, J., J. Tsevat, M. Lave, and J. Roberts (2005). Willingness to pay for a quality-adjusted life year: Implications for societal health care resources allocation. *Medical Decision-Making 27*, 667–677.

Koerkamp, B., M. Hunink, T. Stijnen, J. Hammitt, K. Kuntz, and M. Weinstein (2007). Limitations of acceptability curves for presenting uncertainty in cost-effectiveness analyses. *Medical Decision-Making 27 (2)*, 101–111.

Kruschke, J. (2011). *Doing Bayesian Data Analysis*. Academic Press, Burlington, MA.

Lancaster, T. (2008). *An Introduction to Modern Bayesian Econometrics*. Blackwell Publishing, Oxford, UK.

Laplace, P. (1774). Mémoires sur la probabilité des causes par les évènemens. *Mémoires de mathématique et de physique presentés à l'Académie royale des sciences, par divers savs et lûs dans ses assemblées 6*, 621–656.

Laplace, P. (1812). *Thorie Analytique des Probabilités*. Veuve Courcier, Paris, France.

Lean, M., J. Mann, J. Hoek, R. Elliot, and G. Schofield (2008). Translational research: From evidence-based medicine to sustainable solutions for public health problems. *British Medical Journal, 337*.

Lee, P. (2004). *Bayesian Statistics, 3rd edition*. Arnold, London, UK.

Lindley, D. (1972). *Bayesian Statistics, A Review*. SIAM, Montpelier, VT.

Lindley, D. (1985). *Making Decisions (2nd edition)*. John Wiley & Sons, London, UK.

Lindley, D. (2000). The philosophy of statistics. *The Statistician 49*, 293–337.

Lindley, D. (2006). *Understanding Uncertainty*. John Wiley & Sons, New York, NY.

Loomes, G. and L. McKenzie (1989). The use of QALYs in health care decision making. *Social Science and Medicine 28*, 299–308.

Luce, B. and A. O'Hagan (2003). *A Primer on Bayesian Statistics in Health Economics and Outcome Research*. Bayesian Initiative in Health Economics and Outcome Research.

Lunn, D., D. Spiegelhalter, A. Thomas, and N. Best (2009). The BUGS project: Evolution, critique and future directions. *Statistics in Medicine 28(25)*, 3049–3067.

McIntosh, E., P. Clarke, E. Frew, and J. Louviere (2010). *Applied Methods of Cost-Benefit Analysis in Health Care*. Oxford University Press, Oxford, UK.

Meltzer, M. and S. Teutsch (1998). Setting priorities for health needs and managing resources. In D. Stroup and S. Teutsch (Eds.), *Statistics in Public Health: Quantitative Approaches to Public-Health Problems*. Oxford University Press, New York, NY.

Metropolis, N., A. Rosenbluth, M. Rosenbluth, A. Teller, and E. Teller (1953). Equations of state calculations by fast computing machines. *Journal of Chemical Physics 21(6)*, 1087–1092.

Miller, K. and S. Homan (1994). Determining transition probabilities: Confusion and suggestions. *Medical Decision-Making 14*, 52–58.

Mood, A., F. Graybill, and D. Boes (1993). *Introduction to the Theory of Statistics.* McGraw-Hill, New York, NY.

Morris, S., N. Devlin, and D. Parkin (2007). *Economic Analysis in Health Care.* John Wiley & Sons, Chichester, UK.

Mortimer, D. and L. Segal (2007). Comparing the incomparable? A systematic review of competing techniques for converting descriptive measures of health status into QALY-weights. *Medical Decision-Making 28*, 66–89.

Neal, R. (2003). Slice sampling. *Annals of Statistics 31(3)*, 705–767.

Negrín, M. and F. Vàzquez-Polo (2008). Incorporating model uncertainty in cost-effectiveness analysis: A Bayesian model averaging approach. *Journal of Health Economics 27*, 1250–1259.

NICE (2008). *Guide to the Methods of Technology Appraisal.* National Institute for Health and Clinical Excellence, London, UK.

NICE (2011). *Our Guidance.* National Institute for Health and Clinical Excellence, London, UK.

Nixon, R. and S. Thompson (2005). Incorporating covariate adjustment, sub-group analysis and between-centre differences into cost-effectiveness evaluations. *Health Economics 14*, 1217–1229.

Ntzoufras, I. (2009). *Bayesian Modelling Using WinBUGS.* John Wiley & Sons, New York, NY.

Oakley, J. (2009). Decision-theoretic sensitivity analysis for complex computer models. *Technometrics 51(3)*, 121–129.

Oakley, J. and A. O'Hagan (2004). Probabilistic sensitivity analysis of complex models: A Bayesian approach. *Journal of the Royal Statistical Society B 66(3)*, 751–769.

O'Brien, B. and A. Briggs (2002). Analysis of uncertainty in health care cost-effectiveness studies: An introduction to statistical issues and methods. *Statistical Methods in Medical Research 11*, 455–468.

O'Hagan, A. (1994). *Bayesian Inference, volume 2B Kendall's Advanced Theory of Statistics.* Arnold, London, UK.

O'Hagan, A., C. Mc Cabe, R. Akehurst, A. Brennan, A. Briggs, K. Claxton, E. Fenwick, D. Fryback, M. Sculpher, D. Spiegelhalter, and A. Willan (2004). Incorporation of uncertainty in health economic modelling studies. *Pharmacoeconomics 23*, 539–536.

O'Hagan, A. and J. Stevens (2001). A framework for cost-effectiveness analysis from clinical trial data. *Health Economics 10*, 303–315.

O'Hagan, A. and J. Stevens (2003). Assessing and comparing costs: How robust are the bootstrap and methods based on asymptotic normality? *Health Economics 12*, 33–49.

O'Hagan, A., J. Stevens, and J. Montmartin (2000). Inference for the cost-effectiveness acceptability curve and cost-effectiveness ratio. *Pharmacoeconomics 17*, 339–349.

O'Hagan, A., J. Stevens, and J. Montmartin (2001). Bayesian cost effectiveness analysis from clinical trial data. *Statistics in Medicine 20*, 733–753.

O'Hagan, A., M. Stevenson, and J. Madan (2006). Monte Carlo probabilistic sensitivity analysis for patient level simulation models: Efficient estimation of mean and variance using ANOVA. *Health Economics.*

Pareek, M., J. Watson, L. Ormerod, O. Kon, G. Woltmann, P. White, I. Abubakar, and A. Lalvani (2011). Screening of immigrants in the UK for imported latent tuberculosis: A multicentre cohort study and cost-effectiveness analysis. *Lancet Infections Diseases 11*, 435–444.

Parmigiani, G. (2002a). Measuring uncertainty in complex decision analysis models. *Statistical Methods in Medical Research 11*, 513–537.

Parmigiani, G. (2002b). *Modeling in Medical Decision-Making.* John Wiley & Sons, New York, NY.

Petrillo, J. and J. Cairns (2008). Converting condition-specific measures into preference-based outcomes for use in economic evaluation. *Expert Review Pharmacoeconomics Outcomes Research 8(5)*, 453–461.

Plummer, M. (2010). JAGS: Just Another Gibbs Sampler. http://www-fis.iarc.fr/~martyn/software/jags/.

Price, M. and A. Briggs (2002). Development of an economic model to assess the cost effectiveness of asthma management strategies. *Pharmacoeconomics 20(3)*, 183–194.

Raftery, A. and S. Lewis (1995). The number of iterations, convergence diagnostics and generic metropolis algorithms. In W. Gilks, S. Richardson, and D. Spiegelhalter (Eds.), *Practical Markov Chain Monte Carlo.* Chapman & Hall, London, UK.

Raiffa, H. (1968). *Decision Analysis – Introductory Lectures on Choices under Uncertainty.* Addison Wesley, Reading, MA.

Raiffa, H. and H. Schlaifer (1961). *Applied Statistical Decision Theory.* Harvard University Press, Boston, MA.

Robert, C. (2001). *The Bayesian Choice - 2nd edition.* Springer Verlag, New York, NY.

Robert, C. and G. Casella (2004). *Monte Carlo Statistical Methods - 2nd edition.* Springer Verlag, New York, NY.

Robert, C. and G. Casella (2010). *Introducing Monte Carlo Methods with R.* Springer Verlag, New York, NY.

Robert, C. and G. Casella (2011). A short history of Markov Chain Monte Carlo: Subjective recollections from incomplete data. *Statistical Science 26*, 102–115.

Rowen, D. and J. Brazier (2011). *Technical Document 11: Alternatives to EQ-5D for Generating Health State Utility Values.* NICE Decision Support Unit, London, UK.

Rue, H., S. Martino, and N. Chopin (2009). Approximate Bayesian inference for latent Gaussian models using integrated nested Laplace approximations (with discussion). *Journal of the Royal Statistical Society B 71*, 319–392.

Rushby, J. and J. Cairns (2005). *Economic Evaluation.* Open University Press, Maidenhead, UK.

Saltelli, A., S. Tarantola, F. Campolongo, and M. Ratto (2004). *Sensitivity Analysis in Practice: A Guide to Assessing Scientific Models.* John Wiley & Sons, Chichester, UK.

Savage, L. (1954). *The Foundations of Statistics.* Dover Publications, New York, NY.

Sculpher, M., K. Claxton, M. Drummond, and C. McCabe (2006). Whither trial-based economic evaluation for health decision making? *Health Economics 15*, 677–687.

Senn, S. (2003). *Dicing with Death.* Cambridge University Press, Cambridge, UK.

Smith, J. (1988). *Decision Analysis: A Bayesian approach.* Chapman & Hall, London, UK.

Smith, J. (2011). *Bayesian Decision Analysis: Principles and Practice.* Cambridge University Press, Cambridge, UK.

Sonneberg, F. and J. Beck (1993). Markov models in medical decision-making: A practical guide. *Medical Decision-Making 13(4)*, 322–338.

Spiegelhalter, D., K. Abrams, and J. Myles (2004). *Bayesian Approaches to Clinical Trials and Health-Care Evaluation.* John Wiley & Sons, Chichester, UK.

Spiegelhalter, D. and A. Barnett (2009). London murders: A predictable pattern? *Significance 6 (1)*, 5–8.

Spiegelhalter, D. and N. Best (2003). Bayesian approaches to multiple sources of evidence and uncertainty in complex cost-effectiveness modelling. *Statistics in Medicine 22*, 3687–3709.

Spiegelhalter, D., N. Best, B. Carlin, and A. van der Linde (2002). Bayesian measures of model complexity and fit (with discussion). *Journal of the Royal Statistical Society B 64(4)*, 583–639.

Spiegelhalter, D., A. Thomas, and N. Best (2002). *WinBUGS version 1.4*. MRC Biostatistics Unit, Cambridge, UK.

Stinnett, A. and J. Mullahy (1998). Net health benefits: A new framework for the analysis of uncertainty in cost effectiveness analysis. *Medical Decision-Making 18 (Suppl)*, S68–S80.

Strong, M., J. Oakley, and J. Chilcott (2011). Managing structural uncertainty in health economic decision models: A discrepancy approach. *Journal of the Royal Statistical Society C 61*, 25–45.

Sturtz, S., U. Ligges, and A. Gelman (2005). R2WinBUGS: A package for running WinBUGS from R. *Journal of Statistical Software 12*(3), 1–16. http://www.jstatsoft.org.

Su, Y. and M. Yajima (2010). R2jags User manual: A Package to call jags from R. http://www.cran.r-project.org/web/packages/R2jags/R2jags.pdf.

Thomas, A., B. O'Hara, U. Ligges, and S. Sturtz (2012). Package BRugs manual. http://cran.r-project.org/web/packages/BRugs/BRugs.pdf.

Thompson, S. and R. Nixon (2005). How sensitive are cost-effectiveness analysis to choice of parametric distributions? *Medical Decision-Making 14*, 421–428.

van der Gaag, M., A. Stant, K. Wolters, E. Buskens, and D. Wiersma (2011). Cognitive-behavioural therapy for persistent recurrent psychosis in people with schizophrenia-spectrum disorder: Cost-effectiveness analysis. *British Journal of Psychiatry 198*, 59–65.

van Hout, B., M. Gordon, and F. Rutten (1994). Costs, effects and C/E ratios alongside a clinical trial. *Health Economics 3*, 309–319.

van Rossum, L., van Rijn A., A. Verbeek, M. Oijen, R. Laheij, P. Fockens, J. J., E. Adang, and E. Dekker (2011). Colorectal cancer screening comparing no screening, immunochemical and guaiac fecal occult blood tests: A cost effectiveness analysis. *International Journal of Cancer 128*, 1908–1917.

Venables, W. and Smith, D. and The R Development Core Team. *An Introduction to R*. http://cran.r-project.org/doc/manuals/R-intro.pdf.

von Neumann, J. and O. Morgenstein (1953). *Theory of Games and Economic Behaviour. Third Edition.* John Wiley & Sons, New York, NY.

Whittaker, J. (1990). *Graphical Models in Applied Multivariate Statistics.* John Wiley & Sons, New York, NY.

Willan, A. and A. Briggs (2006). *The Statistical Analysis of Cost-Effectiveness data.* John Wiley & Sons, Chichester, UK.

Willan, A., A. Briggs, and J. Hock (2004). Regression methods for covariate adjustment and subgroup analysis for non-censored cost-effectiveness data. *Health Economics 13*, 461–475.

Wonderling, D., A. Vickers, R. Grieve, and R. McCarney (2004). Cost effectiveness analysis of a randomised trial of acupuncture for chronic headache in primary care. *British Medical Journal 328(7442)*, 747–752.

Woodworth, G. (2004). *Biostatistics: A Bayesian Introduction.* John Wiley & Sons, New York, NY.

World Health Organisation. *Definition of Health.* https://apps.who.int/aboutwho/en/definition.html.

Index

9781032477534